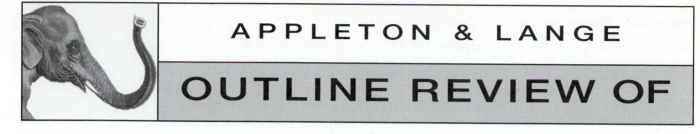

# APPLETON & LANGE

## OUTLINE REVIEW OF

# MICROBIOLOGY & IMMUNOLOGY

D0140604

**William W. Yotis, PhD**

Professor Emeritus of Microbiology
Loyola University Stritch School of Medicine
Clinical Professor of Microbiology and Immunology
University of South Florida College of Medicine
Tampa, Florida

**Appleton & Lange Reviews/McGraw-Hill**
Medical Publishing Division

New York   Chicago   San Francisco   Lisbon   London   Madrid
Mexico City   Milan   New Delhi   San Juan   Seoul   Singapore   Sydney   Toronto

**Appleton & Lange Outline Review of Microbiology & Immunology**

1 2 3 4 5 6 7 8 9 0 CUS/CUS 9 8 7 6 5 4 3

ISBN 0-07-140566-6

This book was set in New Baskerville by Circle Graphics.
The editor was Catherine A. Johnson.
The production supervisor was Sherri Souffrance.
Project management was provided by Columbia Publishing Services.
Von Hoffmann Graphics was the printer and binder.

This book is printed on acid-free paper.

**Library of Congress Cataloging-in-Publication Data**
Yotis, William W.
    Appleton & Lange outline review of microbiology & immunology / William W. Yotis.
        p. ; cm.
    Complement to: Appleton & Lange's review of microbiology & immunology / William
W. Yotis, Herman Friedman, 4th ed. c2001.
    Includes bibliographical references and index.
    ISBN 0-07-140566-6 (alk. paper)
        1. Medical microbiology—Examinations, questions, etc. 2. Immunology—Examinations,
questions, etc. I. Title: Outline review of microbiology & immunology. II. Title: Appleton
and Lange outline review of microbiology and immunology. III. Yotis, William W.
Appleton & Lange's review of microbiology & immunology. IV. Title.
    [DNLM: 1. Microbiology—Examination Questions. 2. Microbiology—Outlines. 3.
Allergy and Immunology—Examination Questions. 4. Allergy and Immunology—Outlines.
QW 18.2 Y66ab 2003]
QR46. Y678 2003
616.9′041′076—dc22
                                                                    2003059955

ISBN 0-07-121981-1 (International Edition)
Copyright © 2004. Exclusive rights by The McGraw-Hill Companies, Inc. for
manufacture and export. This book cannot be re-exported from the country to which it is
consigned by McGraw-Hill. The International Edition is not available in North America.

# Contents

**CHAPTER 3    MEDICAL BACTERIOLOGY**

**CHAPTER 4    MEDICAL VIROLOGY**

## CHAPTER 5    MEDICAL MYCOLOGY

## CHAPTER 6    MEDICAL PARASITOLOGY

# Contributors

**Kenneth E. Ugen, PhD**
Associate Professor of Microbiology and
  Immunology
University of South Florida College of Medicine
Tampa, Florida

**Susan Pross, PhD**
Associate Professor of Microbiology and
  Immunology
University of South Florida College of Medicine
Tampa, Florida

**Sharon Hymes, MD**
Associate Professor of Dermatology
University of Texas Medical School
Houston, Texas

**Nicholas Legakis, MD**
Professor and Chairman of Microbiology
University of Athens School of Medicine
Athens, Greece

# Preface

The plethora of new information in medical microbiology and immunology, while rich and exciting, finds students asking what they have to know in order to pass a qualifying examination in medical microbiology and immunology. The desire to assist medical students or allied health personnel faced with this situation has served as the springboard for the production of *Appleton & Lange Outline Review of Microbiology & Immunology*. The purpose of this book is to provide a rapid, current, and comprehensive review of the relevant information of medical microbiology and immunology. Serious attempts have been made to cover principles and facts of medical microbiology and immunology. This book is targeted for individuals who will be sitting for the USMLE Step 1, State Board, or other medical microbiology and immunology examinations. Because this publication is produced as a complement to our fourth edition of *Appleton & Lange's Review of Microbiology & Immunology,* in contrast to other review books, it adheres to the description of specific, updated topics listed in the recent guidelines of USMLE Step 1. It provides subject-by-subject review for focused attention where it is needed most in general microbiology, medical immunology, bacteriology, virology, mycology, and parasitology to provide valuable assistance for good performance on course examinations and on the USMLE Step 1.

# Basic Microbiology of Infectious Agents 1

*William W. Yotis, PhD*

## I. TAXONOMY OF MICROORGANISMS

### A. Main Differences Between Eukaryotic and Prokaryotic Cells

The human race is subjected to numerous infections caused by bacteria, viruses, fungi, protozoa and metazoa (helminths). Only the helminths are placed within the animal kingdom. The protozoa and fungi are classified in the kingdom of protists. The fungi, protozoa and helminths have more complex cellular organization than bacteria and are eukaryotic. Bacteria are distinguished from plants and animals by their relatively simple prokaryotic cellular organization. Viruses are not considered cells because they depend on other living cells for their multiplication. Table 1-1 lists the main differences between prokaryotic and eukaryotic cells.

### B. Nomenclature and Classification of Microorganisms

Usually each species of a microorganism is assigned an official Latin binomial, with a capitalized genus followed by an uncapitalized species designation. This name is printed in italics. Example: *Staphylococcus aureus*.

### C. Microbial Properties Usually Employed for Classification

1. Cellular composition: DNA, RNA base sequence, protein profiles, fatty acid composition, antigenic composition
2. Shape, arrangement of cells, size, capsule, spore formation, pigmentation
3. Motility
4. Stain reactions (Gram stain, acid fast stain or others)
5. Presence of characteristic surface macromolecules (antigenic structure, phage susceptibility)
6. Metabolic activities
   a. Optimal temperature for growth (mesophilic bacteria grow best at 37°C)

1

► table 1-1

MAIN FEATURES OF PROKARYOTIC AND EUKARYOTIC CELLS

| Cell Component | Prokaryotic Cell | Eukaryotic Cell |
| --- | --- | --- |
| Peptidoglycan in cell wall | + | − |
| Nuclear membrane | − | + |
| Intracytoplasmic membrane | mesosome | endoplasmic reticulum |
| Golgi apparatus | − | usually + |
| Mitochondrion | − | + |
| Microtubule | − | + |
| Flagellum | +/−; simple | +/−; complex |
| Sterols in membrane | − | + |
| Ribosome size | 70s | 80s |

  b. Requirement for, and tolerance to, $O_2$ (aerobic, facultative anaerobic, or anaerobic)
  c. Energy-yielding mechanism (heterotrophic, autotrophic)
  d. Formation of specific metabolic products
  e. Nutritional requirements and abilities to utilize various sugars or other foods
  f. Pathogenicity in animals

## II. CYTOLOGY OF THE BACTERIAL CELL

### A. Major Bacterial Shapes

  1. Spheres (cocci) 0.3–1.0 µm in diameter. Examples include *Diplococcus* (Fig. 1-1), *Streptococcus* (Fig. 1-2) and *Staphylococcus* (Fig. 1-3).
  2. Rods (bacilli) 0.7–10 µm long. Examples include *Bacilli* (Fig. 1-4), *Coccobacilli* (Fig. 1-5), fusiform bacilli (Fig. 1-6), filamentous rods (Fig. 1-7) and curved rods (vibrios, campylobacteria) (Fig. 1-8).
  3. Spirochetes (spiral forms) 4–30 µm long. Examples include *Treponema* (Fig. 1-9), *Leptospira* (Fig. 1-10) and *Borrelia* (Fig. 1-11).

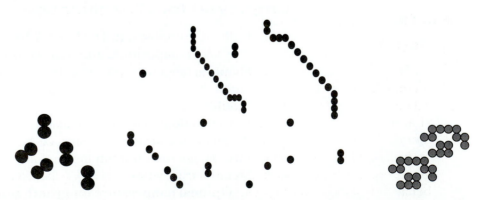

Figure 1-1. *Diplococcus.*  Figure 1-2. *Streptococcus.*  Figure 1-3. *Staphylococcus.*

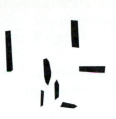
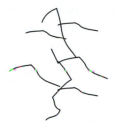

Figure 1-4. *Bacilli.*

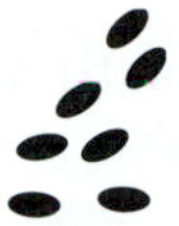

Figure 1-5. *Coccobacilli.*

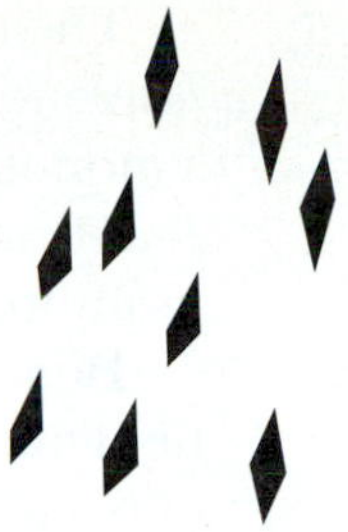

Figure 1-6. Fusiform bacilli.

Figure 1-7. Filamentous rods.

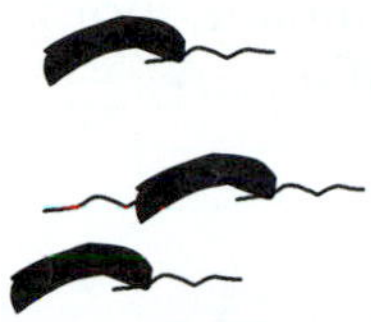

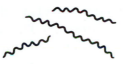

Figure 1-8. Curved rods (vibrios, campylobacteria).

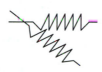

Figure 1-9. *Treponema.*

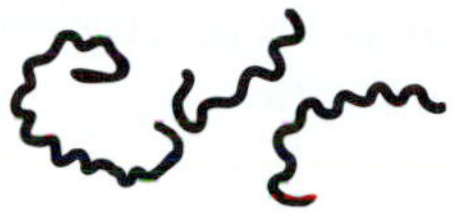

Figure 1-10. *Leptospira.*

Figure 1-11. *Borrelia.*

## B. Surface Layers

### Capsules:

They have the following characteristics.
1. Usually are composed of polysaccharides. Exception: *Bacillus anthracis,* which is composed of D-glutamic acid.
2. Serve as virulence factors because they inhibit phagocytosis.
3. Are used for vaccine production against pneumonia, meningitis and other diseases.

## C. Surface Appendages

### 1. Flagella

Flagella are organs of locomotion. Structurally they consist of a filament, a hook and a basal body. These subunits are composed of proteins called flagellins. Flagellins are immunogenic, species specific and contain H antigens, which are used for diagnostic purposes. The thrust for the motion of bacteria is derived from counter-clockwise rotation of the basal body applied to the filament and driven by the proton motive force. Flagella respond to attractant and repellent substances. This chemotactic behavior is associated with the methylation and demethylation of few cell membrane proteins.

The numbers and distribution of flagella are used for the identification and classification of certain bacteria. For example, *Vibrio cholerae* is a monotrichous bacterium, that is, it contains one flagellum at one pole; *Proteus vulgaris* is a peritrichous organism, that is, it contains flagella over its entire surface.

Demonstration of flagella can be made by electron microscopy, dark-field microscopy, the hanging-drop technique, flagella stain and growth of bacteria in semisolid nutrient agar.

### 2. Pili (Fimbriae)

Pili are hair-like appendages composed of protein called pilin. They can be of two antigenically distinct types. The first type is called common pili. These pili are abundant, short and play an important role in the colonization of epithelial surfaces.

## D. Cell Wall

Cell walls are composed of a continuous peptidoglycan layer that is found in all prokaryotic cells except bacteria belonging to genus *Mycoplasma*. The bacterial cell wall maintains the shape of bacteria, interacts with the components of host defense, plays a role in cell division and is used for serological identification. Enzymes that synthesize cell wall are targets for antibiotics. The cell wall composition is believed to be responsible for the purple staining of Gram-positive bacteria and the red staining of Gram-negative bacteria. The thick peptidoglycan layer of Gram-positive cells greatly hinders the extraction of the crystal violet–iodine complex by acetone–alcohol that is used in Gram staining, and thus Gram-positive cells appear purple. The outer layer of the cell wall of Gram-negative bacteria contains lipids, and the inner layer of peptidoglycan is thin. Thus, the application of acetone–alcohol readily extracts the crystal violet complex from the cell wall of Gram-negative bacteria, which then assume the color of the red counterstain safranin.

### 1. Cell Wall of Gram-Positive Bacteria

Two key components constitute the cell wall of Gram positive bacteria: peptidoglycan and teichoic acid.

a. **Peptidoglycan.** This polymer is composed of many layers of β1–4-*N*-acetylmuramyl-*N*-acetylglucosamine, with side chains of tetrapeptides. The fourth amino acid, D-alanine, is usually directly cross-linked to the ε-amino group of lysine on a neighboring tetrapeptide (penicillin prevents this cross-linking). Figure 1-12 illustrates the structural arrangement of peptidoglycan. Lysozyme cleaves the β1–4 glycosidic bond between *N*-acetylmuramic and *N*-acetylglucosamine. Complete removal of cell wall from Gram-positive bacteria with lysozyme in the presence of an osmotic stabilizing substance, such as sucrose, leads to production of protoplasts. Incomplete removal of cell wall from bacteria results in the formation of spheroplasts. Lysozyme is an antibacterial enzyme found in human tissues and secretions.

b. **Teichoic Acid.** Teichoic acid is a polymer of either ribitol, or glycerol linked by phosphodiester bonds. This polymer is covalently linked to peptidoglycan, has an overall negative charge and can sequester cations from the culture medium for nutritional and metabolic needs.

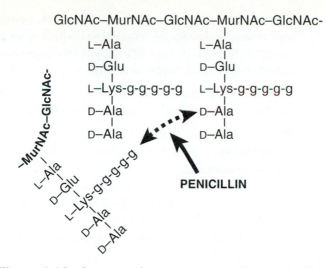

Figure 1-12.  Structural arrangement of peptidoglycan.

## 2. Cell Wall of Gram-Negative Bacteria

The general composition and structure of the wall of Gram-negative bacteria are shown in Fig. 1-13. It is composed of an outer membrane, which is located outside a thin peptidoglycan layer. The outer membrane is basically a bilayered phospholipid structure, and its inner leaflet resembles the composition of the cytoplasmic membrane. The outer leaflet has a unique component called lipopolysaccharide (LPS), or endotoxin. LPS consists of three moieties:

a. **Lipid A.**  This is the toxic moiety of endotoxin. It has been associated with fever, hypotension, shock, death, leukopenia, hypoglycemia, activation of the C3a and C5a components of the alternative pathway of

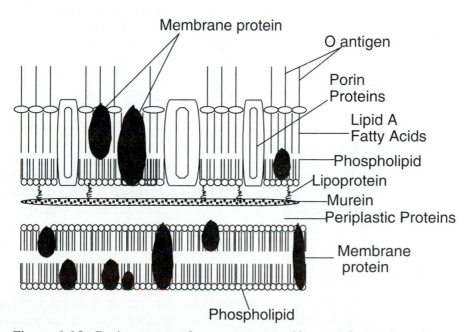

Figure 1-13.  Basic structural arrangement of bacterial cytoplasmic membrane.

complement, induction of interleukins, tumor necrosis factor and gamma interferon. LPS can also induce disseminated intravascular coagulation (DIC) by activation of Hageman factor, resulting in thrombosis, rash, tissue ischemia and damage.

b. **Core.** This consists of series of sugars which include the unique carbohydrates ketodeoxyoctooic (KDO) and heptose.

c. **Specific side chain.** This is a long carbohydrate chain known as the O antigen, which is used for serological identification of Gram-negative bacteria.

Two important proteins are also found in the outer membrane of Gram-negative bacteria. These are the porins which form channels for the entrance of small (molecular weight 600–700) hydrophilic molecules and the metabolite and iron-binding proteins. Finally, the outer membrane serves as a permeability barrier, inhibiting the entrance of certain antibiotics or preventing the loss of periplasmic proteins, such as hydrolytic enzymes including β-lactamase, and sugar, amino acid or iron-binging proteins.

## E. Cytoplasmic Membrane

The cytoplasmic membrane contains 40% lipid and 60% protein. Sterols are found in the eukaryotic cells of fungi, protozoa and helminths, but not in the bacterial membrane. The only prokaryotic cells that contain sterols in their cytoplasmic membrane are the members of the genus *Mycoplasma*. Structurally, bacterial cytoplasmic membranes resemble the lipid bilayer of eukaryotic membranes. The functions of cytoplasmic bacterial membrane include (1) active transport of nutrients, (2) energy production, (3) secretion of toxins and enzymes, (4) biosynthesis of phospholipids, peptidoglycan, LPS, capsular or slime layer (loose capsule) polysaccharides and other macromolecules, (5) attachment of DNA for its replication and separation, and (6) flagellar rotation and chemotactic sensing.

The bacterial cytoplasmic membrane also has medical importance in relation to pathogenicity of such post-streptococcal diseases as rheumatic fever and glomerulonephritis.

A structure very closely related to bacterial cytoplasmic membrane is the mesosome. This cellular component is an invagination of the bacterial cytoplasmic membrane that serves as the origin of the transverse septum that separates the cell in half.

## F. Bacterial DNA

The bacterial DNA consists of a single double-stranded, continuous, circular molecule of DNA. It is not enclosed within a nuclear membrane, and it is devoid of introns, or histones. It contains the genetic determinants controlling the properties of bacterial cells. The haploid genes of bacterial DNA are located in a single chromosome.

## G. Plasmids

Plasmids are extrachromosomal, circular, double-stranded molecules of DNA, which usually replicate independently of the bacterial chromosome (R or resistance plasmids), but they can be incorporated into the bacterial chromosome (fertility plasmids F, F′). The R plasmids play important roles in conferring resistance to antibiotics, antiseptics and ultraviolet light. Fertility plasmids (F, F′) are involved in the transfer of DNA from a donor bacterial to a recipient bacterial cell by conjugation.

## H. Transposons

Transposons are segments of DNA that can move easily inside or between the DNAs of bacteria, bacteriophages and plasmids. In contrast to plasmids, they cannot replicate independently. However, they can replicate as segments of the recipient host cell DNA.

## I. Ribosomes and Polyribosomes

The bacterial eukaryotic ribosomes and polyribosomes (polysomes) contain approximately 60% RNA and 40% protein. The sedimentation constant of ribosomes is 70*s*, and they are composed of two moieties: a 50*s* and a 30*s* subunit. The function of ribosomes is protein synthesis. They are the targets of action of such antibiotics as aminoglycosides, tetracyclines, erythromycin, clindamycin and chloramphenicol.

## J. Spores

Spores are produced intracellularly by members of the genera *Bacillus* and *Clostridium*. Only one spore is produced by a bacterial cell. Each spore contains an exosporium and coat (keratin-like protein), a cortex composed of peptidoglycan and a relatively dehydrated core containing dipicolinic acid and all other bacterial cytoplasmic components. Because of their high resistance to heat, chemicals, desiccation and radiation, bacterial spores play an important role in the survival of certain bacteria and are the source of infectious diseases such as tetanus, gas gangrene, botulism and anthrax. Spore resistance to adverse environmental conditions is thought to be due to the presence of dipicolinic acid, which is found only in bacterial spores.

## III. BACTERIAL NUTRITION

### A. Medical Importance

Diagnosis of various diseases requires cultivation and isolation of the causative agents on culture media that satisfy the nutritional needs of microbes.

### B. Nutritional Types of Microbes

#### 1. Parasites

These can live on dead and living plant or animal tissue. Most pathogenic bacteria are parasites.

#### 2. Obligate Parasites

These microbes can live only on living tissue. Examples: *Treponema pallidum, Mycobacterium leprae,* viruses, rickettsia, chlamydia.

### 3. Saprophytes

Microbes that can live only on dead tissues. These organisms are nonpathogenic.

### 4. Heterotrophic

Microbes that cannot use $CO_2$ as their sole source of carbon. Pathogenic bacteria fit in this group. They obtain energy from the oxidation of organic compounds.

### 5. Autotrophic

Microbes that can use $CO_2$ as their sole source of carbon. They are nonpathogenic and derive their energy from the oxidation of inorganic compounds.

### 6. Auxotroph

Microbes that need nutrients that the parental (prototrophs) types normally synthesize.

## C. Specific Nutritional Requirements

### 1. $H_2O$

It is the universal solvent.

### 2. Carbon

For most pathogenic bacteria, glucose, or at least a two-carbon containing compound, is needed for the production of energy and synthesis of cellular organic macromolecules.

### 3. Nitrogen

Most Gram-positive and Gram-negative pathogenic bacteria require nitrogen in the form of amino acids. Some enteric bacteria can use $NH_4$ as a source of nitrogen.

### 4. Sulfur

Most pathogenic bacteria require an organic source of sulfur usually in the form of methionine or cysteine to synthesize their cellular sulfur-containing macromolecules.

### 5. Oxygen

Bacteria are classified as obligate aerobes, microaerophilic, obligate anaerobes and facultative anaerobes. With the exception of obligate anaerobes, $O_2$ serves as the terminal $H_2$ acceptor. Furthermore, obligate anaerobes lack cytochromes, catalase and superoxide dismutase, which converts the toxic superoxide radical $2O^-_2$ and $2H^+$ to $H_2O_2$. Hydrogen peroxide, which can be lethal, is degraded by catalase of aerobic, microaerophilic or facultative anaerobic bacteria to $O_2$ and $H_2O$.

Obligate anaerobic bacteria are cultured in thioglycolate medium, in anaerobic chambers or in jars containing $H_2-CO_2$ generating systems.

### 6. Growth Factors and Cations

Table 1-2 shows the growth factors and Table 1-3 the cations that are usually added to microbial culture media either when a microbe cannot synthesize them or when they are needed in larger than trace concentrations.

► table 1-2

### GROWTH FACTORS AND CATIONS

| Growth Factor | Function |
|---|---|
| Thiamin | Decarboxylation of keto acids |
| Nicotinic acid; riboflavin | Hydrogen transfer |
| Vitamin $B_6$; pyridoxal | Decarboxylation, deamination, transamination and racemization of amino acids |
| Pantothenic acid (part of CoA) | Acyl activation and transfer, fatty acid synthesis |
| p-Aminobenzoic acid (part of folic acid) | 1-carbon transfer |
| Biotin | $CO_2$ fixation; fatty acid synthesis |
| Vitamin $B_{12}$ | 1-carbon transfer; synthesis of deoxyribonucleosides |

► table 1-3

### KEY CATIONS IN METABOLISM

| Key Cation | Function |
|---|---|
| Mg | In carbohydrate metabolism, stabilization of ribosomes, for amino acid assimilation, for the activation of the $C_1$ and $C_4$ components of complement. |
| Ca | For electrostatic attraction, and penetration of viruses to host cells, for spores, for proteinase activity. |
| P | Required for energy transfer, it is a component of ATP, NAPD, FP, FAD, for the synthesis of nucleic acids and the formation sugar and lipid intermediates. |
| Mn | For enzyme activation, for phosphorylation, for spore formation. |
| Fe | For the formation of cytochromes, catalase, peroxidase, riboflavin, for the production of diphtheria exotoxin. |

## D. Transport of Nutrients Into the Bacterial Cell

There are four main mechanisms by which nutrients enter the bacterial cell: diffusion, facilitated diffusion, active transport and chemiosmotic transport. The key features of these transport systems are shown in Table 1-4.

## E. Bacterial Metabolism

The vast majority of biochemical reactions are the same in individuals, mice and microbes. Slight metabolic differences in human and microbial cells are used to design chemotherapeutic agents to treat infections caused by microbes.

### Carbohydrate Catabolism

Glucose is a major metabolic fuel, and glycolysis (fermentation) is the conversion of sugars to pyruvate without regard to metabolic pathway. The Embden–Meyerhof (EM), hexose monophosphate shunt (HMP), and the Entner–Doudoroff (ED) pathways are the major glycolytic routes. Most cells use EM and HMP at the same time. The ED pathway is not found in animal or plant cells.

When oxygen is present, pyruvic acid produced by fermentation is further metabolized by the tricarboxylic acid cycle (Krebs' cycle), which

► table 1-4

### KEY MECHANISMS OF NUTRIENT TRANSPORT

| Transport Mechanism | Key Features |
|---|---|
| 1. Passive diffusion | Movement of solute from higher to lower concentration. Carrier proteins or energy are not required. |
| 2. Facilitated diffusion | Similar to passive diffusion, but a carrier protein (permease) in cell membrane is needed to transport the solute into the cell to establish equilibrium. |
| 3. Active transport | Permease and energy are needed, solute levels within the cell exceed those found outside the cell. Solute may or may not be altered during transport. It is only altered during the phosphoenolpyruvate (PEP) transport system. |
| 4. Chemiosmotic transport | This is an active transport system which involves the hydrolysis of ATP by ATPase. It is accompanied by the expulsion of protons and the creation of an electrochemical gradient which serves as the driving force for the transport of nutrients. |

produces much more energy in the form of ATP than the glycolytic cycle. This explains why facultative anaerobic bacteria grow rapidly in the presence of oxygen.

Bacteria use the EM, HMP, ED and Krebs' cycle to form some of the basic subunits of proteins, polysaccharides, lipids and nucleic acids.

The production of, or the inability to form, certain end-products or enzymes and the ability or inability to use certain compounds as carbon or amino acid sources are used for the identification of bacteria. For example, *Salmonella typhi* and *Shigella dysenteriae* cannot use lactose as a carbon source, while *Escherichia coli* can; *Staphylococcus aureus* produces coagulase while *Staphylococcus epidermidis* does not. When physiological reactions are used to classify bacteria, it should be noted that variations in these reactions have been observed and such reactions are of doubtful taxonomic value.

## F. Bacterial Culture Media

The diagnosis of bacterial diseases depends upon the isolation and identification of the etiological agents. Isolation of bacteria may be successful only when suitable clinical specimens, proper culture media and conditions of cultivation are closely followed.

The most common culture media used are nutrient agar, blood agar (nutrient agar + blood), or chocolate agar (nutrient agar + heated blood to inactivate antibacterial serum components), cultured at 37°C, in the presence and absence of oxygen. In addition to these, clinical laboratories employ selective and differential culture media. A medium is selective if it inhibits undesirable bacteria and allows desired microbes to grow. Examples of selective media are tellurite agar and Thayer–Martin agar, which are used for the isolation of *Corynebacterium diphtheriae* and *Neisseria gonorrhoeae*, respectively.

A culture medium is differential when biochemical reactions take place in the medium and are indicated by an easily recognizable manner, such as pH indicators or release of certain dyes. These media are employed for the diagnosis of enteric pathogens. A good example of a differential medium is MacConkey agar which is used to separate enteric bacteria into lactose fermentors (*Escherichia coli, Klebsiella pneumoniae, Enterobacter aerogenes*) and nonlactose fermentors (*Salmonella typhi, Shigella dysenteriae, Pseudomonas aeruginosa, Proteus vulgaris*).

## IV. BACTERIAL GROWTH

The usual connotation of bacterial growth is that of an increase in the number of cells, that is, multiplication. This rise in the number of cells occurs by a process called binary fission and involves a transverse division of each cell into two equal cells. There is no mitosis in bacteria. DNA replication occurs continuously, and completion of a round of DNA replication is required for cell division to occur. The replication of bacterial DNA is semiconservative (one strand of the DNA serves as a template for the synthesis of the second, complementary strand) and bidirectional. A bacterial cell in a proper environment grows until it almost doubles its size and then divides by binary fission. During cell division each bacterium forms a new cell wall across its short axis transversely and breaks apart into two daughter cells. Division starts with ingrowth of the cytoplasmic membrane, formation of a complete transverse septum, cleavage and separation. Differences in septum formation and separation are responsible for variation in bacterial shape and cellular arrangements.

Under optimal conditions of growth many bacteria cells divide once every approximately 20–30 minutes. The time required for bacterial cell division is called generation time and is equal to the time elapsed over the number of generations. For example if a cell has divided 4 times within 80 minutes, the generation time is 20 minutes. Some bacteria have long generation times and must be cultivated for weeks to isolate them from clinical specimens. *Mycobacterium tuberculosis* has a generation time of more than 24 hours, thus it requires 2–3 weeks to be isolated from sputum or other clinical specimens. On the other end of the generation time spectrum, *Escherichia coli* divides every 20 minutes, and thus large numbers of cells are produced in a short time. For example, 500 cells of *E. coli* in a urine sample will become 256,000 in 3 hours: 1000 in 20 minutes, 2000 in 40, 4000 in 60, 8000 in 80, 16,000 in 100, 32,000 in 120, 64, 000 in 140, 128, 000 in 160 and 256, 000 in 180 minutes, respectively.

### A. Measurement of Bacterial Growth

#### 1. Determination of Viable Cells in a Urine Specimen by Plate Counts

A measured volume of a diluted sample of urine is spread onto nutrient agar, and following incubation at 37°C of the nutrient agar plates for 16–24 hours the number of bacterial colonies that develop are counted. Each viable cell ideally should give rise to a colony. Assuming that the urine sample has been diluted 1000 times and 100 colonies developed on the nutrient agar plates from a 0.1-mL urine sample, then the number of viable cells per mL of urine sample will be $1000 \times 100 \times 10$, or $1 \times 10^6$ *E. coli* cells. Bacterial counts of $1 \times 10^5$ or more per mL urine indicate a urinary tract infection.

### 2. Determination of the Total Number of Bacteria

Dead and living bacterial cells can be determined by the use of the Petroff-Hauser counting chamber or the use of the electronic Coulter counter.

### 3. Determination of Bacterial Cell Mass

The bacterial cell mass can be determined quickly by turbidimetric or gravimetric analysis.

## B. Bacterial Growth Curve

A generalized bacterial growth curve is shown in Fig. 1-14. It consists of the lag, logarithmic, stationary and death phases.

### 1. Lag Phase

There is no multiplication during this phase of growth. The cells synthesize the required metabolic intermediates for subsequent cell division, and metabolic activity per cell is enhanced due to its increase in size.

### 2. Exponential Phase

During this phase there is an exponential rate of increase in the number of cells and any structural component. It is also in this phase that the cells are most sensitive to antibiotics, heat or low temperatures. For best results the Gram stain should be performed with bacterial cells taken from the exponential phase of growth. The exponential phase stops because nutrients are exhausted and toxic compounds accumulate. Addition of nutrients and removal of toxic metabolic products can maintain bacteria in the exponential phase. The chemostat and the turbidostat are two devices that can be used to maintain bacterial cells in exponential phase.

The quality of a culture medium can be determined by an evaluation of the growth rate $(R)$, which is simply the slope of the growth curve,

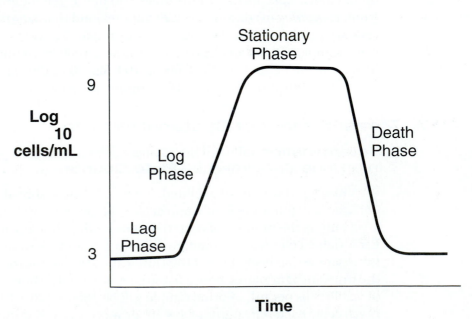

Figure 1-14.  Bacterial growth curve.

determined from the exponential phase. For example, if the number of bacteria increased from 10,000/mL to 100,000/mL in 100 minutes, the growth rate is (100,000 − 10,000)/100, or 900 cells/minute.

### 3. Stationary Phase

This phase of growth is due to drastic reduction of nutrients and the accumulation of toxic metabolic products. During this phase, the rate of cell division is equal to cell death. The number of viable cells remains constant, while the number of dead cells increases. Synthesis of inclusion bodies such as glycogen granules, polyphosphates, or spores may occur in some genera.

### 4. Death Phase

During this phase, bacterial cells die at an almost exponential rate. Some bacteria survive for a very long time due to release of nutrients from cells which die or lyse.

## C. Factors That Influence Bacterial Growth

### 1. pH

Most pathogenic bacteria require a hydrogen ion concentration around 7.0.

### 2. Oxygen Tension

Obligate aerobic bacteria, such as *Mycobacteriun tuberculosis,* require an atmosphere of 20% $O_2$; facultative anaerobic bacteria can grow at $O_2$ atmospheres of 0.2–20%; obligate anaerobes are killed by $O_2$.

### 3. Temperature

Most pathogenic bacteria are mesophilic, that is, they grow best at 35–37°C.

### 4. Osmotic Pressure

Pathogenic bacteria grow best in isotonic media (0.85% NaCl). Hypertonic media cause bacteria to shrink their cell protoplasm (plasmolysis). Hypotonic media cause bacteria to swell their cell protoplasm, and the cell may burst like a balloon (plasmoptysis).

## V. BACTERIAL GENETICS

The genetic material in bacteria is a single, circular molecule of DNA consisting of two long chains of nucleotides. Each nucleotide consists of one phosphate group, one pentose in RNA (or deoxypentose in DNA) and one purine (adenine or guanine) or one pyrimidine (cytosine, thymine or uracil). First, substitution of nucleotides in DNA can lead to silent mutation (does not change the amino acid), missense mutation (changes the amino acid) or nonsense mutation (premature termination of protein synthesis). Second, gene changes can occur by frameshift mutations (mutilated amino acid sequences). Third, mutations can occur when transposons are inserted in the DNA. Fourth, mutations can be induced by chemicals, such as alkylating agents, nitrous acid,

5-bromouracil, and benzpyrene, by radiation with x-rays and ultraviolet light and by phage Mu.

There are four main mechanisms by which bacteria exchange DNA: transformation, transduction, conjugation and transposon insertions. The first three occur between bacterial cells, and the fourth occurs within such cells. Rapid exchange of genetic elements is of immense public health importance in terms of the development of highly virulent and antibiotic resistant bacteria.

## A. Transformation

This mechanism of exchange of DNA involves the simple uptake of deoxyribonucleic acid by bacteria, that is, a dead donor cell lyses and releases its DNA in the environment. A living recipient cell then takes it and incorporates a portion into its own chromosome, which may result in a genetic alteration. Transformation requires a correct ratio of DNA to cells, appropriate cell density, appropriate phase of growth (usually exponential is best) and formation of transformation proteins, for the uptake and incorporation of DNA. It is an uncommon and inefficient mechanism of DNA exchange in bacteria.

## B. Transduction

Transduction is a process in which a bacteriophage carries a piece of bacterial DNA from one bacterial cell to another.

Bacteriophages are composed of an hexagonal head, a neck and tail fibers. The head contains a protein coat, called capsid, and DNA or RNA. The neck contains a central hollow tube and an outer sheath. The tail fibers and the neck are composed of proteins. The tail fibers bind to specific receptors on the bacterial cell surface. This process is called adsorption. The hollow tube then passes through the bacterial cell wall and cytoplasmic membrane. This process is called penetration. Following penetration, the DNA is injected into the bacterial cell cytoplasm. There are two types of phages: the virulent phages, which infect, lyse and kill bacteria, and the temperate or lysogenic phages, which infect bacteria but which do not lyse and kill them immediately. The lysogenic phase DNA, instead of being transcribed, is incorporated into the bacterial DNA. In sharp contrast, the DNA of the virulent phages is transcribed by the bacterial RNA polymerase to messenger RNA (mRNA). New DNA, capsids and enzymes are synthesized. When the bacterial cell is filled with bacteriophages, it lyses and releases phages.

DNA exchange between bacterial cells by transduction can be accomplished by generalized or specialized transduction. In generalized transduction during a lytic infection, bacterial DNA can be accidentally incorporated into the phage instead of phage DNA. This aberrant phage, once released, can still infect other bacteria and inject a segment of the bacterial DNA. The result is transfer of a segment of DNA from one bacterial cell to another by a phage. These are relatively rare events because phages generally take up their own DNA, and any bacterial or plasmid DNA taken up accidentally must be of similar size to phage DNA. Once the DNA transfer has occurred, the likely subsequent transfer of this DNA segment to another cell has the same random chance as the first time.

In contrast to generalized transduction, where random excision and DNA packaging can involve any bacterial gene within the phage DNA, in specialized transduction, which requires a lysogenic phage, only specific genes adjacent to the site of integration within the bacterial DNA are transferred.

## C. Conjugation

This is the most efficient mechanism of DNA exchange between bacteria. It involves direct cell-to-cell contact between related or unrelated bacterial cells, and it is the main mode for the transfer of antibiotic resistance in bacteria.

The conjugal process between cells is controlled by a plasmid called a fertility, or F, plasmid, which contains the genes required for the synthesis of the sex pilus or conjugation tube. The sex pilus is in essence the bacterial penis. Bacterial cells that have F plasmids are designated as F+ cells, or DNA donor male cells, while those that do not have F plasmids are called F− or DNA recipient female cells. The sex pilus penetrates the female F− cell, establishing an opening for the transfer of plasmid DNA to F− cell, the F+ DNA is cleaved enzymatically and one strand of F+ DNA is transferred into the F− cell. Following synthesis of the complementary strand in the F+ and F− cells, the female F− cells are converted to male F+ cells.

Like lysogenic phages, occasionally F+ plasmids of donor bacterial cells can be inserted into the genome of the donor cells. The cells are called Hfr, or high frequency, recombination cells. Now the whole bacterial genome can be transferred to a recipient cell.

The inserted F+ plasmid may excise itself from the genome of male donor cells, carrying with it chromosomal genes. Such plasmids are called F′ (F prime) plasmids.

## D. Transposons

These mobile genes usually transfer genetic information within a DNA donor cell. Even though transposons may lack DNA homology, they can insert genes into bacterial, phage and plasmid DNA. By being able to move into plasmid DNA of diverse bacterial genera, they can alter the antibiotic sensitivity spectra of bacteria, the bacterial pathogenic attributes or other antigenic and metabolic microbial characteristics.

# VI. ANTIBIOTICS

## A. Important Terms

### 1. Synergism

Indicates that a combination of antibiotics X and Y yields a microbial cell count/mL that is smaller than that achieved by either antibiotic X or Y used alone.

### 2. Antagonism

Antagonism between antibiotics X and Y is indicated when the combination of antibiotics X and Y yields a microbial cell count/mL that is higher than that achieved by either antibiotic X or Y used alone.

### 3. Indifference

This term refers to the inability of antibiotic X to alter the antimicrobial properties of Y and *vice versa*.

### 4. Addition

Addition refers to an additive antimicrobial action between antibiotics X and Y.

### 5. Narrow and Broad Spectrum Antibiotic

A narrow spectrum antibiotic is one that is effective against a limited range of microbes, e.g., penicillin G. A broad spectrum antibiotic is effective against a wide range of microbes, e.g., tetracycline.

### 6. Minimum Inhibitory Concentration (MIC)

It is the lowest antibiotic concentration/mL that inhibits the growth of a particular microorganism. It is usually determined by the tube dilution method. The inhibition of growth does not kill the microbes, because removal of the antibiotic allows microbes to grow.

Antibiotics that arrest microbial growth are called bacteriostatic, while those that produce a progressive lethal action and cause a reduction in the number of viable microbial cells are called bactericidal.

### 7. Antibiotic Resistance

Ordinarily refers to genotypic changes that persist during further cultivation in the absence of an antibiotic. Thus a penicillin resistant *Staphylococcus* derived from a strain that was originally sensitive to penicillin is considered penicillin resistant. An enteric bacterium never sensitive to penicillin is considered nonsusceptible rather than resistant.

### 8. Cross Resistance

When a microbe is resistant to two or more related antibiotics at a time, it shows cross resistance, e.g., a microbe resistant to tetracycline also shows resistance to most of the other modified tetracyclines.

## B. Key General Rules for Clinical Use of Antibiotics

1. Clinical specimens must be taken prior to initiation of antimicrobial therapy. If antimicrobials have been used prior to taking a clinical sample, microbes most likely will not be isolated.
2. The possible allergic or other adverse effects of antimicrobials should always be considered prior to their administration.
3. Effective use of antibiotics requires suitable dosage and period of administration.
4. A smear and a Gram or other suitable stain of infected body fluids or exudates often provide an immediate guide to specific antimicrobial therapy.
5. Prophylactic chemotherapy is not indicated for respiratory illness. Approximately 95% of such illness is not caused by bacteria but probably by various viruses. Attempts to use antibiotics to prevent complications caused by secondary bacterial infections are contraindicated; antibiotics should be used only after a secondary infection has been established. The

indiscriminate use of antibiotics has promoted the development of antibiotic resistance in many microbes.

6. In serious or life-threatening infections, bactericidal rather than bacteriostatic antimicrobials must be used. Furthermore, the bactericidal antimicrobials must be administered intravenously rather than orally or intramuscularly.

## C. Mechanism of Action of Antimicrobial Agents

### 1. Cell Wall Inhibitors

a. **The Penicillin Group.** This group of antibiotics includes the following: (a) chemically unmodified penicillins (benzyl penicillin, phenoxymethylpenicillin and phenoxyethyl penicillin); (b) aminopenicillins (ampicillin, hetacillin, amoxicillin); (c) penicillinase resistant penicillins (methicillin, oxacillin, nafcillin, cloxacillin, dicloxacillin); (d) antipseudomonal penicillins, which include the carboxypenicillins (carbenicillin, imipenem), the ureido and piperazine penicillins (mezlocillin, azocillin and piperacillin) and the monobactams (aztreonam); (e) cephalosporins, which include the first-generation cephalosporins (cephalothin, cephapirin, cephradine, cefazolin), the second-generation cephalosporins (cefamandole, cefoxitin) and the third-generation cephalosporins (cefotaxime, moxalactam).

All of the antibiotics listed in the penicillin group possess a β-lactam ring and are known as β-lactams.

The β-lactam ring is the site of action of penicillinase (β-lactamase), yielding the inactive product penicilloic acid.

b. **Mode of Action of β-Lactams.** The β-lactams enter the bacterial cell through porins, bind to penicillin binding proteins (PBPs) on the outside of the cytoplasmic membrane and prevent further cross-linking of the cell wall peptidoglycan. Specifically, β-lactam prevents the transpeptidation reaction linking the carboxyl group of the terminal D-alanine on the tetrapeptide to the amino group of the neighboring pentapeptide cross-link. This is the primary action of a β-lactam. The secondary action involves the activation of such peptidoglycan hydrolases as amidase and muraminidase, which cause loss of integrity of peptidoglycan, and lysis of the bacterial cell.

Resistance to β-lactam antibiotics for Gram-positive bacteria is the result of production of β-penicillinase, which destroys the carbon–nitrogen bond in the β-lactam ring of the penicillin molecule. Gram-negative bacteria can become resistant to β-lactam drugs either by production of β-lactamase or by alteration of the porins of the outer membrane of their cell wall, thus inhibiting the entry of β-lactams into the bacterial cell layers. Finally, resistance of either Gram-positive or Gram-negative bacteria to β-lactam antibiotics can be due to alterations in the penicillin-binding proteins.

Most antibiotic resistance arises from a chromosomal mutation, acquisition of a plasmid or a transposon.

c. **Other Cell Wall Inhibitors**

i. ***Vancomycin.*** Vancomycin is a glycopeptide that inhibits peptidoglycan chain elongation by binding directly to the D-alanyl-D-alanine moiety of the peptidoglycan pentapeptide, while the β-lactam antibiotics bind transpeptidase. Vancomycin is used as a second-line antibiotic for the treatment of serious *S. aureus* infections that are resistant to penicillinase resistant antibiotics, e.g., nafcillin. It is also the drug of choice when the patient is intolerant to penicillins and cephalosporins. Vancomycin has a common property with the penicillin group of antibiotics in that it is bactericidal.

Microbes can become resistant to vancomycin when the normal binding site of vancomycin D-alanine-D-alanine changes to D-alanine-D-lactate.

### ii. Bacitracin and Cycloserine.
Bacitracin inhibits dephosphorylation of the 55-carbon lipid carrier undecaprenol pyrophosphate to phosphate. It is too toxic for parenteral use, and it is employed as an ointment for the superficial skin infections. Cycloserine is a competitive antagonist for D-alanine, inhibiting two reactions: the racemate that forms D-alanine from L-alanine and the enzyme that forms D-alanyl-D-alanine dipeptide. Cycloserine is used as a second-line antibiotic for the treatment of tuberculosis. Both bacitracin and cycloserine are bactericidal drugs.

### iii. Isoniazid, Ethambutol, Ethionamide.
These three drugs are active, bactericidal cell wall inhibitors used for the treatment of mycobacterial infections. Although the mode of action of these antibiotics has not been completely detailed, it is currently believed that isoniazid and ethionamide interfere with the synthesis of mycolic acid, which is a constituent of the mycobacterial cell wall. Ethambutol interferes with the synthesis of a cell wall polysaccharide called arabinogalactan.

Resistance to isoniazid is due to a mutation of the peroxidase-catalase gene, while resistance to ethambutol is due to an alteration of the arabinosyl transferase gene.

## 2. Antibiotics Affecting the Cytoplasmic Membrane

a. **Polymyxins.** These are cyclic, bactericidal polypeptide antibiotics that affect Gram-negative bacteria, especially *Pseudomonas*. Polymyxins act like detergents, inserting themselves within the cytoplasmic membrane and causing leakage of vital cellular components. Because polymyxins are very toxic to the kidneys, they can be used only externally for the treatment of such localized infections as eye infections, skin infections and external otitis media.

b. Antifungal Antibiotics

i. **Nystatin and Amphotericin B.** These drugs have long ring structures with many double bonds in the macrolide ring, and they are known as polyene antibiotics. Nystatin and amphotericin B bind specifically to ergosterol of the fungal cytoplasmic membrane. This binding causes leakage of intracellular $K^+$. Further damage to fungal membrane induces leakage of amino acids, nucleotides and other larger intracellular molecules, culminating in the eventual death of the fungal cell. Amphotericin B is the drug of choice for systemic fungal infections, including candidiasis. Where oral or topical therapy for *Candida albicans* infection is indicated, nystatin is preferable to amphotericin B. Both of these drugs are toxic to the kidneys. The nephrotoxicity of amphotericin B may be reduced by enclosing the antifungal agent within lipid spheres called liposomes.

ii. ***Azole Drugs.*** This group of antifungal agents includes the imidazoles (ketoconazole, miconazole, clotrimazole) and the triazoles (fluconazole, itraconazole). Ketoconazole, fluconazole and itraconazole are commonly used for such systemic infections as candidiasis, cryptococcosis, histoplasmosis, coccidioidomycosis, blastomycosis, chromoblastomycosis and invasive aspergillosis. Miconazole and clotrimazole are very toxic and are used topically for such fungal infections as dermatophytosis, cutaneous candidiasis, vaginitis and pityriasis versicolor. The azole antifungal drugs inhibit the synthesis of ergosterol by stopping the methylation of lanosterol, which is a precursor of ergosterol. Bacterial cells do not have ergosterol in their cytoplasmic membrane, while the mycoplasmal, or human cell, membrane contains cholesterol, and thus the synthesis of their sterols when present cannot be expected to be compromised.

## 3. Antibiotics Affecting Protein Synthesis

### a. Drugs Acting on the 30s Portion of Bacterial Ribosome

i. ***Aminoglycosides:*** Gentamicin, Tobramycin, Streptomycin, Amikasin, Neomycin, Aminocyclitol, Spectinomycin. These antibiotics are bactericidal and have selectivity for Gram-negative aerobic bacteria and some acid-fast microbes. Extensive research with streptomycin indicates that aminoglycosides destroy bacteria by causing misreading of messenger RNA and interruption of protein synthesis (inhibition of initiation complex), that is, in susceptible bacteria they pass through the cell wall, the cell membrane and cell cytoplasm and bind irreversibly to the 30s ribosomal proteins. This attachment leads to production of abnormal proteins due to misreading of messenger RNA and termination of protein synthesis due to early detachment of ribosomes from messenger RNA.

Use of aminoglycosides may cause nephrotoxicity and damage to the vestibular and auditory moieties of the eighth cranial nerve.

The most common mode by which bacteria become resistant to aminoglycosides is enzymatic acetylation, adenylation or phosphorylation of the amino and hydroxyl groups of these drugs. In the case of enterococci, antibiotic resistance to aminoglycosides is due to reduced drug uptake, while in pseudomodal species drug resistance is due to alteration of the bacterial ribosome.

Low pH, high salts and anaerobic conditions present in septic foci, such as abscesses, or in the urinary tract limit the action of aminoglycosides. Active transport of aminoglycosides into the bacterial cell requires aerobic conditions, which is why anaerobes are resistant to aminoglycosides.

Spectinomycin is closely related to aminoglycosides and may be used to treat gonorrhea caused by penicillin resistant strains of *Neisseria gonorrhoeae*.

*ii. **Tetracyclines:*** Doxycycline, Minocycline, Oxycyclin. These antibiotics are bacteriostatic for Rickettsia, Chlamydia, Mycoplasma, Brucella, Borrelia and other selected Gram-positive and Gram-negative bacteria. Tetracyclines block the binding of the aminoacyl transfer RNA to the acceptor site of the 30$s$ subunit of the bacterial ribosome.

Resistance to tetracyclines stems from the active efflux of the drugs out of the bacterial cell.

Use of tetracyclines has been associated with permanent staining of teeth of children less than 9 years old, enamel hypoplasia, depression of bone growth and suppression of normal enteric flora leading to diarrhea and overgrowth of drug resistant microbes.

### b. Drugs Affecting the 50s Moiety of Bacterial Ribosome

*i. **Chloramphenicol.*** This antibiotic is bacteriostatic for most microbes that are susceptible to its action but bactericidal for *Hemophilus influenzae, Neisseria meningitidis* and *Streptococcus pneumoniae.* Its antibacterial spectrum extends to Gram-positive and Gram-negative bacteria, rickettsia and chlamydia. An undesirable aspect of chloramphenicol is its toxicity that may lead to aplastic anemia. To avoid its well-known toxicity it is necessary to monitor the serum level of chloramphenicol and keep it below 50 μg/mL.

Chloramphenicol binds to 50$s$ subunit of the bacterial ribosome and then blocks the activity of peptidyltransferase, i.e., the transfer of the growing peptide attached to a transfer RNA and located on the P site on the 50$s$ subunit of the ribosome. The end result is inhibition of protein synthesis.

Resistance to chloramphenicol may result from acetylation of the drug by an acetyl transferase encoded by genes of a plasmid.

*ii. **Clindamycin.*** This antibiotic is a macrolide that has a mode of action similar to chloramphenicol. However, it is not a broad spectrum drug because it is used primarily for anaerobic bacteria such as *Bacteroides fragilis, Fusobacterium* and other anaerobic organisms associated with intra-abdominal infections. Clindamycin is also used for septic abortions.

*iii. **Erythromycin.*** The antibacterial spectrum of erythromycin is similar to penicillin, but individuals allergic to penicillin are not allergic to erythromycin. It is bacteriostatic and is the drug of choice for *Legionella pneumophila, Campylobacter jejuni* and *Mycoplasma pneumoniae* infections.

Erythromycin binds to 50$s$ subunit of the bacterial ribosome and inhibits the translocation step by blocking the release of the uncharged transfer RNA from the donor site following peptide bond formation. Resistance to erythromycin occurs via modification of the transfer RNA.

## 4. Inhibitors of Bacterial Nucleic Acid Synthesis

### a. Inhibitors of RNA Synthesis

***Rifampin.*** This bactericidal antibiotic is used for the treatment of tuberculosis. A derivative of rifampin called rifabutin is used for prevention of disease caused by *Mycobacterium avium-intracellulare* in immunocompromised patients. The mode of action of rifampin and its derivative is inhibition of the bacterial RNA polymerase which leads to blockage of messenger RNA synthesis. Because rifampin resistant organisms emerge rapidly, this antibiotic is used in combination with other drugs.

b. Inhibitors of DNA Synthesis

*Quinolones:* Ciprofloxacin, Norfloxacin, Ofloxacin, Nalidixic Acid. These antibiotics are effective against both Gram-positive and Gram-negative bacteria. The first quinolone used for urinary bacterial infections, nalidixic acid, has now been replaced by ciprofloxacin due to the rapid resistance that developed against nalidixic acid.

The mode of action of quinolones is inhibition of DNA gyrase, which coils strands of DNA.

DNA gyrase is composed of $\alpha$ and $\beta$ subunits. Quinolones bind to the $\alpha$ subunit of DNA gyrase, and alteration in this subunit is the main mechanism of resistance to quinolones.

c. Inhibitors of the Synthesis of DNA Precursors

i. *Sulfonamides:* Sulfamethoxazole, Trimethoprim. These antibiotics inhibit Gram-positive and Gram-negative bacteria, *Nocardia asteroides, Chlamydia trachomatis* and such microbes as *Toxoplasma gondii, Pneumocystis carinii* and *Isospora belli.*

Sulfonamides resemble *p*-aminobenzoic acid (PABA), which is part of folic acid (FA). The active form of FA is tetrahydrofolic acid ($FH_4$), a coenzyme important in the transfer of one-carbon units required in the synthesis of adenine, guanine and thymine, the key constituents of nucleic acids. Sulfonamides, by inserting themselves in the place of PABA, act as competitive inhibitors of PABA and thus block the synthesis of nucleic acids. Trimethoprim also blocks nucleic acid synthesis by inhibiting the enzyme dihydrofolate reductase. This enzyme converts dihydrofolic acid ($FH_2$) to $FH_4$. The main mechanism of resistance to trimethoprim is acquisition of a plasmid that codes for the formation of trimethoprim resistant dihydrofolate reductase.

Combination of sulfamethoxazole and trimethoprim provides a synergistic action and also reduces the development of resistance to sulfonamides.

Dapsone, used for the treatment of leprosy, and *p*-aminosalicylic acid (PAS), used for the treatment of tuberculosis, also act as competitive inhibitors of folic acid.

# VII. STERILIZATION AND DISINFECTION

## A. Definition

*Sterilization* indicates the elimination of all viable microbes and spores. Disinfection refers to the destruction of pathogenic microbes but not spores. Sterilization or disinfection is generally accomplished by destruction, removal or inhibition of germs by use of physical, mechanical or chemical agents.

## B. Physical Agents

### 1. Moist Heat

Boiling for 2–10 minutes will kill the vegetative forms of pathogenic bacteria and fungi. However, boiling does not usually kill bacterial spores of many pathogenic fungi or certain viruses, such as the hepatitis viruses. This is the simplest method of destroying microbes from objects and materials that are stable to heat.

### 2. Autoclaving (Compressed Steam)

To destroy spores, the temperature must be raised to 121°C. Heating at 15 lb of steam pressure in a chamber called an autoclave will raise the temperature to 121°C. Heating for 20 minutes under these conditions will sterilize small objects.

### 3. Pasteurization

Refers to heating of milk at 60°C for 30 minutes. Pasteurization kills 97–99% of the vegetative microbial cells present and 100% of tubercle bacilli, salmonellae, streptococci, brucellae, listeriae or other microbes that cause milk-borne disease.

Microbial cell destruction at elevated temperatures indicated above is due to denaturation of proteins, e.g., coagulation and hydrolysis, as well as destruction of the cell membrane.

### 4. Dry Heat

It is used to sterilize glassware. Materials in the oven must be maintained at a temperature of 165°C for 120 minutes to destroy all microbes including spores.

### 5. Radiation

Two forms of irradiation may be used to kill microbes: ultraviolet light and x-rays. Ultraviolet rays (260 nm) are absorbed by nucleic acids, producing lethal mutations or major chemical modifications, such as formation of thymine dimers and addition of hydroxyl groups to nucleic acid bases. Exposure of irradiated microbes to sunlight cleaves thymine dimers and reverses the action of ultraviolet light. This phenomenon is called photoreactivation.

Ultraviolet light, unlike ionizing radiation (x-rays), possesses low penetrative power and is only active on smooth surfaces. Furthermore, it can damage the cornea. These limitations have reduced but not eliminated the use of UV light in medicine, because of its well-known bactericidal properties. Figure 1-15 shows the death curve of *Escherichia coli* after exposure to ultraviolet light.

Examination of this death curve (Fig. 1-15) indicates that there is a 90% reduction in the surviving cells for each 30-second exposure. That is, in 30 seconds, the surviving cells were reduced from $10^6$ to $10^5$. The number of viable cells remaining after an additional 30 seconds was reduced to $10^4$ (10,000), and so on.

Ionizing radiation such as x-rays is the product of radioactive decay consisting of $\alpha$-, $\beta$-, and $\gamma$-rays. These rays, especially the $\gamma$-rays, have higher penetrative power and much more energy and lethal ability than ultraviolet light. Therefore, they are used for sterilization of syringes, surgical gloves, plastic items, disposable items, and in the food industry.

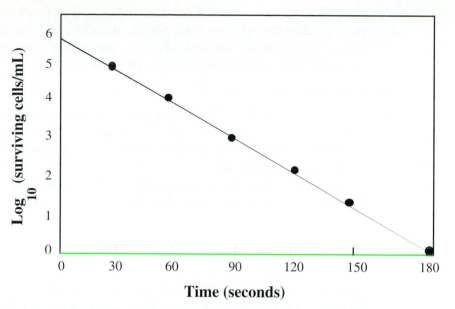

Figure 1-15. Death curve of *E. coli* after exposure to UV light.

The mode of action of ionizing radiation is production of lethal hydroxyl radicals and breakage in the DNA double helix.

## C. Mechanical Agents

### Filtration

Filtration is the main method by which heat-labile biological fluids or liquid bacterial culture media are used to remove bacteria. Routinely used filters are 0.2-μm porous disks composed of biologically inert cellulose esters. Microbial cells or particles larger than 0.2 μm in diameter are retained on the surface of the 0.2-μm pore size cellulose filters. Most viruses are smaller than 0.2 μm and usually pass through these filters.

## D. Chemical Agents

The antimicrobial action of chemical agents is influenced by several factors. First, the concentration of the chemical agent. The antimicrobial action of a substance usually is not a linear function of its concentration. The relationship of the rate of killing of microbes $K$ to the concentration of a substance $C$ and time $t$ is $K = tC^n$, where $n$ is a constant. The value of $n$ may differ between varying antimicrobial substances. Only for substances having a $n$ value of "one" is the rate of antimicrobial action in linear proportion to the concentration of the test substance. With a chemical substance that has an $n$ value of 2, the rate of reaction would be proportional to the square of the concentration, and with an $n$ value of 3, to the cube of the concentration of the antimicrobial agent. Second, as with all chemical reactions the temperature is important and must be specified. Usually for every 10-degree increase in temperature, there is a 2- to 3-fold increase in the rate of antimicrobial action of a chemical agent. Third, as with heat sterilization, organic materials such as proteins combine with antimicrobial agents and reduce their effectiveness. For example, mercuric chloride is an efficient antibacterial agent in water, but in the presence of blood or serum it loses much of its antibacterial action. Fourth, pH can alter the antimicrobial action of a chemical agent. In general, acidity increases the strength of an antimicrobial chemical substance, especially phenol or chlorine-containing compounds.

## 1. Oxidizing Agents

Iodine, chlorine and hydrogen peroxide are the most useful disinfectants. Chlorine is employed as a water disinfectant, and iodine as a skin disinfectant. Calcium hypochloride in 1–5% solution is an excellent agent to disinfect solid surfaces.

The mode of action of oxidizing agents is inactivation of enzymes by changing functional sulfhydryl (HS) groups to nonfunctional S–S groups.

## 2. Detergents

These compounds possess a water-soluble anion or cation (hydrophilic) and a long-chain lipid soluble (hydrophobic) group. The hydrophobic group inserts itself in the microbial membrane, while the hydrophilic group positions itself in the surrounding medium. The net result is release of small vital metabolites from the microbial cell and interference with active transport of nutrients due to reduction of interfacial tension. This is why detergents are called surface active agents. Benzalkonium chloride is a cationic detergent used frequently for skin disinfection.

## 3. Alcohols

Ethyl alcohol (70%) is widely used as a disinfectant; 0.2% iodine in 70% ethanol is an excellent germicidal, but not sporocidal, agent.

Alcohols remove lipids from microbial membranes and thus alter their structure and function. They also denature cellular proteins.

## 4. Phenols

These compounds sold under the trade name of Lysol are now used for disinfection of floors, toilets and other surfaces. Phenols disrupt cytoplasmic membranes and denature cellular proteins.

## 5. Alkylating Agents: Formaldehyde, Glutaraldehyde and Ethylene Oxide

These compounds are used to sterilize respiratory therapy equipment. The mode of action of formaldehyde, glutaraldehyde and ethylene oxide is addition of alkyl groups ($CH_2$) to OH or $NH_2$ groups of microbial proteins and nucleic acids.

# Immunology 2

*Kenneth E. Ugen, PhD*

## I. INTRODUCTION

We are constantly being exposed to foreign substances in our environment, and it is the job of the immune system to provide us with protection. Therefore, the most important function of the immune system is to protect an individual or organism from infection and disease caused by microorganisms including primarily bacteria, viruses, fungi and protozoa.

### A. Definitions and Major Components of Immunity

#### 1. Immunity

Reaction to and protection from foreign (i.e. non-self) substances in the environment. The foreign substances are known as antigens, and these include microbes, tumor antigens and external proteins as well as polysaccharides.

#### 2. Immune Response

Mobilization of effector cells and humoral factors which interact with antigens and eliminate them from the body.

#### 3. Immunogen/Antigen

Chemical or substance that is foreign to the host which when injected into the host induces an immune response.

#### 4. Innate and Acquired Immunity

Innate immunity occurs very rapidly and is usually not dependent on specific cellular and humoral immune responses but is dependent mainly on natural barriers. In contrast, acquired immunity is dependent mainly on specific immune responses mediated by cellular and soluble humoral factors. Unlike innate immunity, acquired immunity develops over time and is not immediate.

## II. INNATE IMMUNITY

Intact skin provides an initial, major, powerful barrier against infection. In addition, the fatty acids released by the sebaceous glands of the skin have antibacterial as well as antifungal activity, which is important for mediating innate immunity. Likewise, the ciliated mucosa of the epithelium lining of the respiratory tract provides some nonspecific protection from infection as well as the extreme acidity of the stomach. Some of the other innate immune mechanisms include pattern recognition receptors (PRR), acute phase proteins, as well as phagocytic and natural killer cells. Examples of PRR include lipopolysaccharide-binding proteins, collectins, complement proteins, defensins and the more recently identified and characterized Toll-like receptors. Another important "player" in innate immunity is the complement system which will be described later in this chapter.

## III. ACQUIRED IMMUNITY

This type of immunity differs from innate immunity in that it involves cells of the immune system called lymphocytes, immunomodulatory molecules called lymphokines, antibodies, as well as killer T cells. Adaptive immunity can function on its own with certain antigens, but the majority of the effects are mediated through the important interactions between antibody and the complement and the phagocytic cells associated with innate immunity. This type of immunity is divided into active (through natural infection and vaccination) and passive (i.e. transplacental and serum therapy).

### A. Humoral and Cellular Immunity

Humoral immunity utilizes predominantly antibodies, i.e. called antibody mediated immunity. Cellular immunity utilizes killer T lymphocytes and phagocytes, i.e. cell mediated immunity. The soluble mediators of acquired immunity other than antibodies are as follows.

#### 1. Lymphokines, Cytokines, Chemokines

These are produced by a number of cells of the body and overall are important in regulating the immune system and other myriad important responses in the body. Examples of this class of soluble mediator include the interleukins (IL), the interferons (IFN), as well as tumor necrosis factor (TNF).

#### 2. Acute Phase Proteins

These are induced by stress and participate in inflammatory processes and healing. Examples of acute phase proteins include the C reactive proteins.

#### 3. Complement

The complement system is a critical component of the immune system, is activated by immune complexes and has important roles in the regulation of immunity. Complement entails a serum cascade system that is composed of over 20 proteins.

## B. Consequences of Immune Activation

In general, activation of the immune system can have a number of consequences, some of which are beneficial and others being detrimental. The major ones are as follows.

### 1. Phagocytosis

The ingestion of particles by macrophages and neutrophils.

### 2. Inflammation

A series of processes or reactions that brings cells and other mediators of immunity to the site of infection and damage. It involves an increase in vascular permeability and migration of lymphocytes.

### 3. Neutralization

Involving, in general, the combination of an antibody with an antigen usually as part of an infectious agent and the resultant inactivation of the pathogen.

### 4. Cytotoxic Reactions

Utilizing various types of killer cells that can interact with target cells (i.e. either cells infected with various infectious agents or tumor cells) and kill them.

## C. Cells and Tissues of Immunity

The major types of cells that are involved in immunity are granulocytes, macrophages and lymphocytes. These cells originate in the hematopoetic cells in the bone marrow. In a functional sense these different types of cells differ in their contribution to the immune system. They can perform effector functions such as antibody secretion and cytokine release as well as killer cell function and phagocytosis. The cells can also have important functions in the regulation of the immune system including the release of important immunomodulatory cytokines. White blood cells are relatively short-lived cells that need to be constantly renewed. In this renewal process immature lymphocytes become educated in "primary" organs to respond to foreign (i.e. non-self antigens); these "educated" lymphocytes then are transferred to secondary lymphoid tissues, i.e. the spleen and lymph nodes, where they are then selected by antigen.

### 1. Lymphocytes

These are small cells which are found in blood, lymph and other tissues especially lymphoid tissue. They exist as different subtypes, i.e. as B cells, T helper cells (Th1 or Th2 (i.e. type 1 and type 2), which secrete different cytokines), cytotoxic T cells (Tc), T suppressor cells (Ts), as well as natural killer (NK) cells. The subtypes are phenotypically defined by different cell surface (i.e. CD markers) which are expressed on the surface of the cells.

a. **T Lymphocytes.** These cells display certain CD markers, some of which have functional significance. In addition, they express antigen specific T cell receptors (TCR). Some display the α/β TCR type, which constitutes the majority of cells, while others display the γ/δ type, which has more restricted expression. CD4 surface expressing T cells are helper cells (Th1/Th2) that mainly produce cytokines which regulate immunity. CD8-expressing T cells are usually cytotoxic cells that typically perform "killer" functions. The figure below shows the general structure for the α/β T cell receptor (TCR) consisting of the two (α and β) chains consisting of the variable ($V_\alpha$ and $V_\beta$) and constant ($C_\alpha$ and $C_\beta$) regions (Fig. 2-1).

b. **B Lymphocytes.** These cells also typically display certain CD markers as well as antigen specific B cell receptors (BCR). B cells can present antigen to T cells as well as produce antibody (i.e. as differentiated plasma cells) and cytokines under the influence of T cells.

c. **Natural Killer Cells.** These types of cells can display certain CD markers but do not possess a definable antigen specific receptor. They can recognize and destroy virus-infected cells and tumor cells that have lost the self-antigen "signature." NK cells also kill by antibody-dependent cellular cytotoxicity (ADCC) and regulate immunity by cytokine secretion.

d. **Mononuclear Phagocytes.** These cells are somewhat larger than lymphocytes and have various functions including phagocytosis and clearance of microbes and cellular debris, wound healing and repair, antigen presentation and immune regulation through cytokine secretion. They contain a number of cell markers and receptors for complement, antibodies, as well as for immunomodulatory cytokines.

e. **Antigen Presenting Cells (APCs).** These important components of the immune system comprise a wide range of different cell types that, overall, have a high concentration of MHC class II molecules. The major types of antigen presenting cells are Langerhans cells in the skin, follicular dendritic cells in the lymph nodes, interdigitat-

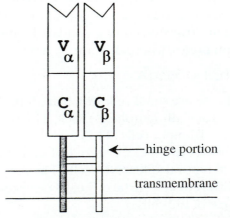

Figure 2-1.  Basic structure of a T cell receptor.

ing cells in the thymus, as well as B cells and macrophages. Their important role is to process and present antigen to T lymphocytes, which is necessary for activation.

f. **Polymorphonuclear Granulocytes.** These are amoeboid and granular cells. They comprise the majority of leukocytes in the blood, have a relatively short half-life and move from blood to tissues by means of diapedesis. These cells exist as neutrophils (90% in blood), eosinophils (2–5%) and basophils (>1%). The neutrophil can be considered to be an acute phase phagocyte that produces and responds to cytokines. It also releases a number of tissue-destroying enzymes, making them important in host defense against infection. Other examples are basophils as well as tissue mast cells, which have specialized granules containing chemical mediators of allergy and inflammation.

g. **Primary Lymphoid Organs.** The major primary lymphoid organs are the thymus and the bone marrow. These organs are mainly composed of epithelial cells and lymphocytes and provide a micro-environment for "education" and development of lymphocytes.

h. **Thymus.** The thymus is a two-lobed organ within the thoracic cavity which contains thymocytes in various stages of maturity. Importantly, the stem cells from the bone marrow circulate to the thymus, where T cells mature into either $CD4^+CD8^-$ or $CD4^-CD8^+$ T cells. The thymus has a medulla and thymus and contains helper cells, such as thymic epithelial cells, interdigitating cells and macrophages in addition to thymic lymphocytes. The thymus involutes with age as well as with stress.

i. **Bone Marrow.** The bone marrow contains a number of different immature as well as mature cells. It provides an environment for growth of all blood cells including B cells but not T cells.

j. **Spleen.** The spleen is located in the left abdominal quadrant, is composed of lymphocytes, macrophages and reticular fibers and is organized into red and white pulp. The white pulp is enriched with lymphocytes and contains "T and B cell zones" as well as follicles and germinal centers.

k. **Lymph Nodes.** Lymph nodes are located in clusters throughout the body and are composed of lymphocytes, macrophages and reticular fibers and are organized anatomically into cortex and medulla. The cortex is organized into T and B cell zones. In addition to lymphocytes, these zones can contain antigen presenting cells such as macrophages and reticular cells.

## 2. Mucosa-Associated Lymphoid Tissue (MALT)

The MALT are aggregates of lymphoid tissue in the submucosa of the GI, respiratory and GU tracts. They are composed of follicles and germinal centers as well as APCs, B cells and T cells. MALT produces secretory IgA, which has the important role of providing surveillance and protection against infectious agents that enter through the mucosa (i.e. the respiratory and gastrointestinal tracts).

## IV. STRUCTURE OF ANTIGENS AND ANTIBODIES

Antigens (Ag) are foreign substances that induce the formation of antibodies and cell mediated immunity (CMI). Organisms, including humans, have evolved in a worldwide environment filled with antigens, and evolutionarily it has become necessary to become responsive to an almost limitless number of antigenic epitopes. It is clear that most organic macromolecules spanning the gamut from proteins to lipids can function as antigens; however, proteins have been shown to function effectively as the best antigens. The major reason for the better antigenicity of proteins likely deals with the cell machinery that is in place for processing, presenting and recognizing antigen in the immune system, and it favors the handling of proteins over other macromolecules. Antigens have been referred to by various names, such as immunogens (i.e. induces immunity), tolerogens (i.e. induces tolerance) and haptens. Haptens are very small chemical groups that confer antigen specificity on larger carrier molecules. The rank order for immune potential is as follows: proteins > polysaccharides > nucleic acids > lipids with decreasing immunogenicity.

In terms of how antigens are handled and recognized by lymphocytes, it is clear that antigens must be degraded into shorter pieces and then presented by antigen presenting cells to T cells in order for proper activation to take place. This is one of the hallmark principles of how antigens are recognized by T cells. By contrast, and importantly, the antigen receptors on B cells can recognize "native" nonprocessed antigen. The short peptides that are recognized by T cells are generally 9–20 amino acids in length. Complex antigens may have a number of antigenic determinants (i.e. epitopes) and as such are designated to be multivalent. As an example, a 30-kDa protein antigen may have 9–10 distinct epitopes and is then designated as a mixed determinant immunogen.

### A. Factors Affecting Immunogenicity

In terms of producing better, stronger immunity, the more complex an antigen is the better. Also, antigens that are particulate in nature also tend to be better antigens than those that are soluble. Other factors not related directly to the nature of the antigen can significantly affect the immune response. These include, among other things, the route and dose of the antigen. In general, the subcutaneous and intradermal routes of delivery are the best. Other factors, including adjuvants and schedule of inoculation, can also influence the immune response. The immune potential of the animal being injected can also influence the type and extent of the immune response that an animal will mount.

### B. Properties of Immunoglobulins

Serum proteins within the blood are electrophoretically divided into albumins and globulins. Globulins are divided into γ, β, and α globulins. Humans and lower mammals have five classes of immunoglobulin molecules: IgG, IgM, IgA, IgD and IgE, and these belong to the γ globulin fraction of serum proteins. The basic structural unit of antibodies consists of four polypeptide chains, two identical heavy chains (H) of about 50 kDa each, and two identical light chains (L) of about 25 kDa each. Each light chain is disulfide bonded to one H chain, and H chains are disulfide bonded to each other. IgG, IgA, IgD and IgE exist in the blood in this four-chain structure. In addition, IgA and IgM can exist in more complex structures involving 2–4 chain aggregates for IgA and 4–5 chain aggregates for IgM. IgG molecules are divided into four subclasses numbered 1, 2, 3 and 4. IgA is divided into two subclasses, 1 and 2. The classes and subclasses of immunoglobulins are present in serum in defined concentrations and have other known properties, such as serum half-life etc.

## C. Antibody Structure

The two H chains of IgG have unique amino acid sequences that define its class and subclass markers as well as antigen binding capacity and biological function. The H chain contains one variable and three constant domains. A domain is a peptide sequence with motifs of conserved amino acids that confer a common domain structure. IgG also has two light chains (called $\kappa$ and $\lambda$) with one variable and one H chain. The variable domains of H and L have amino acid sequences that are unique from one IgG to the next (hypervariable regions), and it is in these regions of variability that the antibody makes actual contact with the antigen. The variations in the hypervariable regions of the V domains are called idiotypic variations because they vary within a single member of a species. In every human serum are many different types of idiotypes. IgG, IgA and IgD H chains have 3 constant domains while IgM and IgE H chains have four constant domains. All L chains (both $\kappa$ and $\lambda$) have one constant domain. Unique sequences in the H domains allow for isotypic variation (common to all member of the species, i.e. every human contains the same identical isotypes), allotypic variation (variation between members of the species), complement binding, Fc binding and disulfide bond formation. During the assembly process that takes place in B cells each L chain aligns with and attaches to the V domain and first C domain of each H chain. This portion of the molecule is referred to as the Fab portion and contains the antigen binding domains. The remaining domains of the two H chains form the Fc region of the molecule. Receptors for the Fc portion of the antibody molecule reside on a number of cell types. These receptors bind to the Fc portion of the immunoglobulin molecule and mediate engulfment and opsonization of the pathogen bound to the Fab portion of the immunoglobulin. Figure 2-2 shows the basic structure of the antibody molecule including the light and heavy chains, the variable regions on the light and heavy chains ($V_L$ and $V_H$) and the constant regions of the light ($C_L$) and heavy chains ($C_{H1}$, $C_{H2}$ and $C_{H3}$).

## V. COMPLEMENT

The complement system is considered to be the major effector limb of the humoral immune system. It is composed of at least 20 chemically defined serum proteins that interact as an enzyme cascade. The two different pathways constituting the complement system differ in their activation parameters but share a common terminal reaction sequence. Importantly, uncontrolled activation of complement as well as deficiencies of the complement components result in serious disease states. Sequential activation of the components of the complement results in

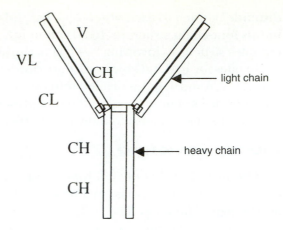

Figure 2-2.  Basic structure of immunoglobulin molecule.

several important activities: (1) the release of inflammatory peptides,
(2) release and deposition of the complement component C3b, which
mediates phagocytosis (i.e. opsonization), and (3) mediation of lysis of
cells through membrane damage.

Two pathways for complement activation have been described. The
first is called the classical pathway. Under normal homeostatic and physiological conditions this pathway is activated by antigen–antibody complexes. The specific antibody types involved in the classical pathway are
IgG and IgM. The antigen–antibody complex leads to the formation of a
convertase, which splits the C3 component of the cascade to produce C3b
which has the central role in both the classical and the alternative pathways. The C3b component is centrally important because it combines with
other components of the complement system to form the membrane
attack complex (MAC), and it also has a role in opsonizing bacteria.
Briefly, in the classical pathway the antigen–antibody complex activates
the C1 component. This, in turn, results in the cleavage of the C2 and C4
components to form the C4b2b complex, which functions as a C3 convertase which cleaves C3 into C3a and C3b. The C3b, in turn, forms a
complex with C4b2b, resulting in the generation of a new enzyme called
C5 convertase. This enzyme cleaves C5 to C5a and C5b. C5b then combines with several other complement components (C6, C7, C8 and C9)
to produce the MAC, which mediates lysis of cells. The alternative pathway is likely to be more ancient from an evolutionary standpoint, and it
is distinguished from the classical pathway mainly because of its lack of
necessity for the C1, C2 or C4 components. Therefore, activation of
the alternative pathway occurs without the need for antibody through an
antibody–antigen interaction. As such a number of different molecules
can initiate C3 conversion. These include components of Gram-negative
and Gram-positive bacteria, fungal and yeast cell walls, tumors as well as
parasites. These components can initiate the alternative cascade pathway
by binding to C3 and another component called factor B. Another component, properdin, functions to stabilize the C3b–B complex. The C3–
factor B complex is then cleaved by a protease called factor D to produce
C3bBb, which acts as a C3 convertase that generates more C3b. A number of receptors and other specific factors have evolved to appropriately
control the complement cascade. These include inhibitors of the C3 and

C5 convertase as well as molecules that inactivate C4b for the classical pathway as well as interfere with the C3bBb complex for the alternative pathway. There are several inherited or acquired complement deficiencies that can result in pathologic conditions. For example, deficiencies in components C5–C8 can increase susceptibility to *Neisseria* bacteremia as well as other infections. Likewise, a deficiency in C3 can result in recurrent and severe infections of the sinus and respiratory tract. Also, because the complement components are synthesized in the liver, individuals with severe liver disease such as alcoholic cirrhosis or chronic hepatitis often cannot synthesize enough complement components and therefore suffer from a higher incidence of infection with pyogenic bacteria.

# VI. ANTIBODY–ANTIGEN INTERACTIONS AND FUNCTIONS

The amino end of the heavy and light chains of antibodies contains discrete hypervariable regions that are responsible for specific binding to antigen. These hypervariable regions are also called complementarity-determining regions (CDRs) and as indicated represent the areas of the molecule that come in contact with the antigen. There are three CDRs in each H and L chain. Importantly the hypervariable regions of the H and L chains come in juxtaposition to form the antigen-binding site or cleft. During this process amino acids on both the antigen and antibody come in close contact with each other and form various non-covalent bonds. The better the fit for the antigenic epitope and antibody-binding cleft, the greater the number and strength of the association. Therefore, the higher the specificity, the higher the affinity is for the antigen. The carboxy ends of heavy and light chains are much less variable but do contain amino acid regions that confer select functions such as complement activation and binding to Fc receptors.

## A. Antibodies Functioning as B Cell Receptors

Antibodies can be secreted as either membrane associated or secreted forms. The membrane forms serve as antigen receptors on B cells (BCR) and result in antigen binding, presentation and B cell differentiation to plasma cells (which are primarily antibody-secreting cells) and memory B cells. The secreted forms of antibody combine with antigen in the extracellular space and result in neutralization of the organism or molecule that expresses that antigen. The membranous forms of immunoglobulins have H and L chains, with the H chains containing a variable region, transmembrane region and cytoplasmic domain. The total BCR complex is similar to the T cell receptor complex in that both are hetero-oligomers containing different chains involved in either binding antigen or signaling cell activation. The immunoglobulin molecule is designed with high affinity and specificity, while the constant region end binds to complement proteins and Fc receptors which promote antigen elimination. IgG is also a primary mediator of ADCC (antibody dependent cellular cytotoxicity). Likewise IgG and IgA are also important in neutralizing pathogens most notably viruses. Both IgG and IgA can neutralize mucosal pathogens, with IgA having a particularly important role.

## B. Humoral Immune Response

   Upon the initial or primary encounter with antigen, the generation of specific antibodies can generally be noted after a lag period of 7–10 days. The initial antibodies to appear are IgM followed typically by IgG, the levels of which decay more slowly than IgM. The secondary immune response refers to an additional encounter with the same antigen up to decades after the initial exposure. In this situation there is a considerably more rapid immune response when compared to the kinetics after the first exposure. The lag phase for the secondary immune response is typically truncated, i.e. 3–5 days in length. This is apparently due to stimulation of "memory" B cells, which are formed after the initial exposure and form the pool of "rapid responders" that are called into action after the secondary immune response. In the secondary response, both IgM and IgG are produced, and IgG is generated at a much higher level than in the primary immune response and lasts considerably longer. With each subsequent exposure to the same antigen, the antibodies generated tend to bind antigen with a higher affinity. This is due to the process of affinity maturation. Affinity maturation results from point mutations occurring within the hypervariable regions of the antibody molecule. Figure 2-3 illustrates diagrammatically the primary and secondary humoral immune responses.

## VII. GENERATION OF ANTIBODY DIVERSITY AND IMMUNOGLOBULIN GENES

   As indicated elsewhere in this chapter, the ability of the immune system to recognize antigens depends on antibodies generated by B cells and on antigen receptors expressed by T cells. In terms of antibodies, a basic question had been how antibodies arise. Two hypotheses had been put forth to explain antibody generation: (1) the "instructional" hy-

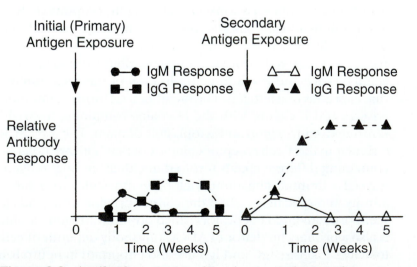

Figure 2-3. Antibody responses in primary and secondary immune responses.

pothesis, wherein the antigen would instruct B cells to make a specific antibody, and (2) the "selectional" hypothesis, whereby an antigen selects a B cell with a predetermined, pre-existing ability to make specific antibody. It is the selectional hypothesis (i.e. clonal selection) that has been shown to be responsible for generating specific antibodies.

Antibodies are the major workhorses of the immune system in terms of mediating protection, either after natural infection or vaccination, against a large variety of pathogens. It can obviously be appreciated that a large antibody repertoire must exist to respond to the diversity of pathogenic antigens to which the body is exposed. It is estimated that for both antibodies and T cell receptors there is $10^6$–$10^9$ different specificities possible. In fact, it is estimated that a person makes more different forms of antibodies than all other proteins in the body combined. This obviously provides a problem if we assume that the concept of "one gene leads to one protein" holds. If one gene is needed to code for each antibody molecule, then certainly most of the genome in human cells would be needed to code for all of the different immunoglobulins needed to respond to the varied antigenic insults to which we are constantly exposed. Clearly this cannot be the case. Fortunately, nature has developed a method to solve this problem. The solution involves having a relatively small number of immunoglobulin genes, which can rearrange and combine with each other to produce the large number of immunoglobulin molecules with the precise antigenic specificities. For this rearrangement process there is a finite set of variable (V) and constant I region genes. Each of the V genes can rearrange and associate with any of the C region genes instead of having one gene encoding for the entire Ig molecule. Rearrangements and reassociations of V and C regions occur for both the heavy and light chains of the immunoglobulin molecules. Additional diversity for Ig molecules is attained with the presence of J (joining) region genes for both heavy and light chains as well as D (diversity) region genes for the heavy chains only. Overall, then, the large diversity present in the antibody repertoire results from DNA rearrangement events as well as RNA splicing. The DNA rearrangement event is catalyzed by recombinases, which are encoded by the RAG-1 and RAG-2 genes (recombination activating genes). The importance of these genes is demonstrated in transgenic mice in which mutations or deletions of these genes show arrest of lymphocyte development as well as severe combined immunodeficiency. Briefly, the process begins with the initial DNA rearrangement within the germline. This step involves excision of some of the gene segments which bring together the specific genes that will be maintained into closer juxtaposition. This is then followed by a transcription step which produces a primary RNA transcript. This is subsequently followed by a splicing step which results in a mature mRNA molecule consisting of a V-J-C (constant) region segment for the light chain and a V-D-J-C (constant) region segment for the heavy chain. These are then translated to produce the respective mature polypeptides. An important concept for the DNA rearrangement process is that the early rearrangement events occur in the absence of antigen. That is, antibody specificity is "selected" by the antigen from a previously determined pool of antibody specificities. Also the specificity of the B lymphocyte is fixed during the variable region gene rearrangement process. Only the "effector" functions of the immunoglobulins produced can be changed through class switching of the constant region genes. In terms of what constant regions are translated in the antibodies produced in the initial immunoglobulins produced, the rule is that the constant region genes that are immediately adjacent to re-arranged VJ or VDJ regions are the ones that are produced. These constant regions genes are for the μ and δ heavy chains, which explains why B cells that express IgM and IgD are the immunoglobulins that are produced first. Class or isotype switching is mediated through switch regions that are immediately 5' to each of the constant region genes. Under appropriate T cell activation signals including cytokines, differing class switching scenarios are signaled. For example, helper factors from T cells in general stimulate a switch to IgG production, whereas specifically IL-4 induces a switch to production of IgE, IL-5 results in the production of IgA, while interferon γ stimulates a switch to IgG3. Again, class switching does not change the specificity of the antibody, which, as indicated above, has been previously determined. It changes only the effector function of the antibody. That is, switching to IgG allows the generation of this important humoral mediator of protection against a wide variety of pathogens. In addition, IgG can cross the placenta and can passively immunize an unborn baby with protective immunoglobulins from the mother. Likewise, switching to IgA results in a secretory immunoglobulin which can neutralize mucosal pathogens. In addition, class switching only occurs in the heavy chains. Overall, the major mechanisms for the generation of antibody diversity are (1) availability of multiple V, J and D gene segments and the recombinatorial associations that can occur among them; (2) random associations between H and L chains; (3) diversity generated at the junctions of the various gene components making up the Ig (this is called junctional diversity, N-region diversification, etc.); and (4) somatic cell mutation, i.e. mutations occurring within the hypervariable region of the Ig molecule that do not affect the specificity of the antibody but which do increase the affinity. Somatic mutation usually occurs during class switching. The scheme for immunoglobulin production is summarized as follows: (1) the process begins with the heavy chain with a recombination between D and J regions; (2) the DJ region then recombines with the V region; (3) the gene sequence VDJ-μ-δ is then transcribed; (4) the VDJ-μ-δ product then functions to stimulate the recombination of the V and J regions of the light chain; (5) this recombined region is then transcribed to produce the mRNA for either the VJ-κ or the VJ-λ light chains; (f) the recombined μ and δ heavy chains as well as the λ or κ light chains are then translated and assembled into the membrane-bound IgM and IgD molecules. Finally, after primary stimulation or exposure to antigen, IgM is secreted, and, following secondary antigen stimulation with T cell help, class switching to IgG, IgA or IgE can occur with the generation of these secreted antibodies.

## VIII.  MAJOR HISTOCOMPATIBILITY COMPLEX (MHC)

The MHC is a region of highly polymorphic genes whose products are involved with recognition of self, recognition of foreign antigens as well as various cell–cell interactions. Another important role of the MHC is to associate with antigen and the T cell receptor which results in T cell activation. In humans the complex consists of the human leukocyte antigens (HLA). They differ among different members of the same species; i.e. they are considered to be alloantigens. HLA-A, HLA-B and HLA-C code for class I MHC proteins while three HLA D loci code for class II MHC proteins, DP, DQ and DR. Virtually all nucleated cells display MHC class I molecules on their surface. The complete class I molecule consists of a 45,000 molecular weight heavy chain complexed to a molecule called $\beta_2$-microglobulin. The heavy chain is highly polymorphic, which is a characteristic important for the recognition of self from non-self. MHC class II molecules are found on the surface of certain cells such as dendritic cells, Langerhans cells, B cells and macrophages. They are highly polymorphic as well and consist of two chains that are linked non-covalently. The MHC class I and II molecules have a centrally important role in immunology since the ability of T cells to recognize antigen is critically dependent on the association of processed antigen with either class I or class II proteins. Generally, cytotoxic T cells and helper T cells recognize antigen in the context of "self" MHC class I and class II molecules, respectively. This is the important concept known as MHC restriction. MHC molecules also have important roles in estimating the likelihood of developing autoimmune diseases as well as the likely success of organ transplants.

The acceptance or rejection of a transplant is, in considerable part, determined by the class I and II molecules on the donor cells. Class II and particularly the DR locus appear to be the most critical. In the so-called graft-versus-host (GVH) response, it is the CD8-positive cytotoxic T cells that mediate most of the cytotoxic killing. Figure 2-4 shows the general structure of the class I and class II MHC molecules.

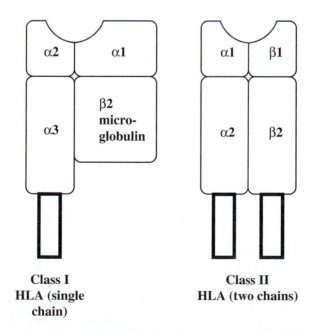

Figure 2-4. General structure of class I and class II major histocompatibility molecules.

## IX. T CELL ACTIVATION

Lymphocyte activation can be considered to be a series of ordered biochemical and molecular processes in which a resting lymphocyte is stimulated to divide and produce progeny that will be specific for a particular antigen. The most important requirement for lymphocyte activation is the specific binding of foreign antigen to T cell receptor proteins. An important characteristic of this process is that the antigens must be processed before they are presented to T cells. Another requirement for full T lymphocyte activation is co-stimulatory responses from antigen presenting cells delivered to the lymphocytes. This, in particular, is a requirement for the processing of monomeric antigens. Therefore, T cells, i.e. helper T cells, recognize processed antigens (approximately 8–12 amino acids in length) only and then only when bound to MHC class II molecules. These antigens are processed within antigen presenting cells (APC) such as macrophages within an endosome where the fragment then becomes associated with MHC class II molecules. The complex then migrates to the surface of the cell, where it can interact with T cells. Evolution has provided a method whereby the binding cleft on the MHC class II molecule is protected from promiscuous binding by nonspecific peptides. This invariant chain binds to the binding cleft on MHC class II molecules. When this complex arrives at the endosome, the invariant chain is degraded, which allows the specific peptide to bind to the cleft for eventual presentation to the T cell. The types of antigens that are presented to helper T cells through association with MHC class II molecules have been designated exogenous antigens. These antigens are usually associated with infectious agents that enter antigen-presenting cells by endocytosis. On the other hand, endogenous antigens such as those from viruses as well as tumor cells are processed by different methods and are typically presented to CD8-positive cytotoxic T cells through MHC class I antigens. These endogenous antigens are likewise cleaved to small peptides but in an organelle called a proteosome. They then become associated with a protein called TAP (transporter associated with antigen processing), which effectively carries the peptide into the endoplasmic reticulum where it becomes associated with the MHC class I protein. This complex then migrates through the Golgi apparatus, where it is subsequently presented on the surface of the APC and presented to cytotoxic T cells. The activation of helper T cells holds a central role in the immune response in that it provides important "helper factors" which are important for cytotoxic T cell activation and effector function as well as for B cell activation. IL-1 released for example by macrophages that function as APCs is necessary for efficient helper T cell activation. In addition to the requisite interaction between processed antigen, MHC and lymphocyte receptors, an additional step is necessary for full activation. This additional step is a co-stimulatory signal provided by the molecule B7.1/B7.2 (CD80/CD86) on APCs which interacts with CD28 on helper T cells. This in turn results in the production of important immunomodulatory cytokines, which are important for proper lymphocyte activation. In most circumstances without this co-stimulatory signal full activation does not occur and anergy (a state of non-responsiveness) occurs. In addition to the antigen–T cell receptor interaction and co-stimulatory molecules, other accessory molecules that mediate adhesive functions also have a role in lymphocyte activation by enhancing interactions between APCs and lymphocytes. These important accessory molecules include LFA-1 on T cells and ICAM-1 on APCs.

## X. B CELL ACTIVATION

It is clear that interactions between T cells and B cells are important for proper B cell activation. This interaction is one of the hallmarks of the functioning of the immune system; i.e. the dependence of a number of important processes of the immunity, including B cell activation, on helper T cell function. The importance of T cell help for B cell activation can best be described in a scenario where the B cell functions as an APC. In this situation antigen will bind to membrane IgM or IgD (mIgM or mIgD) and become internalized through endocytosis. It will then become processed through the exogenous protein processing machinery that has already been described with the processed protein becoming associated with MHC class II molecules. This processed protein–MHC class II complex will then activate, along with appropriate co-stimulation, helper T cells which in turn will produce helper factors, i.e. cytokines (most notably and importantly IL-2), which will stimulate the growth and development of B cells. The full activation of B cells requires two other interactions besides the engagement of antigen with the B cell receptor. These are (a) the interaction of the costimulatory molecule B7 on B cells with CD28 on T cells and (b) the interaction of the CD40 ligand (CD40L) on T cells and CD40 on B cells. The co-stimulatory molecule–CD28 interaction has been indicated above to be necessary for the activation of T cells and the subsequent release of the critical IL-2. The CD40–CD40L interaction has been demonstrated to be required for class switching from IgM to the other effector immunoglobulin isotypes. Defects in this important CD40–CD40L system can result in conditions such as the hyper-IgM immunodeficiency syndrome, in which class switching from IgM to IgG cannot occur, resulting in severely impaired immunity due to a lack of IgG necessary to neutralize a large number of infectious agents. Treatment of babies who have this syndrome is through administration of hyperimmune immunoglobulins containing IgG against the major pathogens affecting the babies.

## XI. CELL-MEDIATED IMMUNITY

Shortly after infection, microbial toxins and antigens induce innate immunity through the release of cytokines and other inflammatory mediators. These can then activate and attract cellular blood elements such as phagocytes, natural killer (NK) as well as platelets to the site of infection. This cellular immune response in general helps to limit the spread of the infection. It also promotes the degradation of microbes to component antigens for transport to the immune organs for activation of adaptive immunity. In terms of innate cellular immunity, microbial antigens, particularly those from bacterial cell walls, activate cells and serum defense mechanisms which are chemotactic for phagocytes and NK cells as well as increase blood accumulation at the site of infection. This limits the spread of infection and degrades microbes for antigen presentation to T cells. The serum factors activated by microbial antigens belong to the complement, kinin and clotting systems. Cells can be activated to release cytokines such as tumor necrosis factor (TNF) and interleukin-12 (IL-12) that also participate in the inflammatory process. When the host immune system is challenged by harmful cellular elements, such as tumor cells, or host cells harboring eukaryotic microbes, such as protozoa and fungi, it responds with killer T cells and macrophages. These immune effector cells attack the harmful cellular elements and destroy them. In order to induce this cell-mediated immunity (CMI), microbial antigens are processed by APCs, presented to T cells and the T cells either regulate other cells or become killer cells. CD4$^+$ helper cells influence either antibody production (TH2) or CMI (TH1). This differential maturation is controlled by the cytokine environment, with IL-12 and interferon $\gamma$ promoting TH1 and IL-4 and IL-10 promoting TH2. Once TH1 cells are activated, interferon $\gamma$ and other cytokines are released and activate macrophages to attack and destroy the target cells. These cytokines can also activate NK cells and CD8$^+$ killer cells. Cytotoxic effector mechanisms involve predominantly CD8$^+$ T cells. These cells, as indicated elsewhere, are MHC class I restricted and become potent killer cells when activated by antigens and cytokines from TH1 cells. Activated CD8$^+$ killer cells bind to target (i.e. virus-infected cells) and release granules called perforin, and these form pores in the membrane of the target cell leading to cell death. When CD8$^+$ expressing T cells become activated, they also express the Fas ligand. This surface-located peptide binds to the Fas antigen on target cells and activates the cellular proteases that mediate apoptosis. Granzymes released from killer cell granules may also contribute to DNA fragmentation. NK cells are activated by TH1 cytokines (LAK cells) to lyse certain tumor and virus targets. Of course NK cells do not express the TCR, therefore, target recognition has been somewhat of a mystery until recently. It now appears that NK cells have receptors for self-MHC class I alleles, and, if these are missing, lysis of the target occurs. NK cells have lytic granules like CD8$^+$ cells and utilize perforin in exactly the same fashion.

Antibody-dependent cellular cytotoxicity (ADCC) as the name implies involves the cooperation of Fc$^+$ killer cells and specific antibodies. Antibodies binding to cell surface antigens on target cells interact with Fc receptors in killer cells, resulting in activation. T cells as well as NK cells and macrophages can participate in ADCC. Macrophages have a much broader array of mechanisms for killing. Upon activation by phagocytosis or inflammatory cytokines, macrophages release a variety of cytokines, enzymes and free radicals, which promote microbial and tissue destruction as well as tissue repair and lymphocyte activation.

## XII.  VACCINES

Vaccines have been one of the truly great success stories of medicine. Through their action against infectious diseases, vaccines have prevented or ameliorated more human suffering that any other medical intervention. Vaccination (derived from the Latin word *vacca*= cow) can be defined as a deliberate attempt to boost immune responses through active immunization with an antigen. This is often called active immunity, and it can often generate protective long-term immunity after a lag period necessary for the active development of immune responses. Passive immunity usually refers to the infusion of preformed antibodies against an antigen from an infectious agent. In this case, immunity is immediate but not long-lasting because of the relatively short half-life of antibodies, which limits how long they will be effective. A good example of passive immunity is the transfer of maternal IgG to the baby. This is important for protecting the baby against infection while its immune system is developing. Another example of life-saving passive immunization or immunotherapy is the treatment of snake bites with horse serum against the toxin.

Another term to define is adoptive immunity. This term usually refers to the passive transfer of immune cells rather than antibody into animals for the purpose of imparting passive cellular immunity. In making a vaccine, an initial dilemma must be overcome; that is, to separate the two effects of disease-causing organisms. This entails isolating or creating an organism, or a portion of one, that is not able to cause full-blown disease but still retains the antigens responsible for inducing host immune responses.

## A. Major Types of Vaccines

A number of different types of vaccine strategies are available with associated advantages and disadvantages.

### 1. Live Attenuated Vaccine

For a number of viral and bacterial pathogens the live attenuated vaccine is, in principal, the ideal type of preparation for a vaccine because it will replicate at a low level and will usually be very strongly immunogenic. Also, as it will usually infect cells, it will be processed as an endogenous as well as exogenous protein. As such it will stimulate cytotoxic T cell activity as well as T helper cell responses and antibodies. A potential disadvantage of this type of vaccine preparation is the potential for reversion of attenuation. This would cause an infection, which would result in the very disease that the vaccine is meant to prevent. Live attenuated vaccines can be particularly problematic in immunosuppressed individuals, children and the elderly. An example of a live attenuated vaccine is the oral (Sabin) polio vaccine.

### 2. Killed Vaccine

The killed or inactivated vaccine preparation consists of an organism or portion of organism which has been killed or inactivated by some treatment (i.e. formalin, heat, $\gamma$ irradiation etc). Although these types of preparations have a better safety profile than live attenuated vaccines, they induce a more limited immune response because they are unable to undergo any type of replication that would normally effectively drive both humoral and cellular immune responses.

### 3. Toxoid Vaccine

The toxoid vaccines are toxins that are treated with or absorbed with aluminum salts. In these cases an adjuvant usually needs to be added to increase the immunogenicity. Examples of toxoid vaccines include diphtheria and tetanus toxoids, which are usually combined with an acellular pertussis vaccine which functions as a vaccine on its own as well as providing an adjuvant effect for diphtheria and pertussis.

### 4. Subunit Vaccine

This type of vaccine includes peptide vaccines or recombinant protein vaccines that are generated by DNA cloning technologies. Peptides as vaccines have some advantages since one can present specific immunogenic epitopes in a relatively small preparation, thus maximizing the development of immune responses to these areas. Disadvantages of peptide vaccines include a lack of conformationality for the epitope that occurs in an intact recombinant protein that may be important for immunogenicity. Recombinant protein vaccines created by recombinant DNA technology have also been used for pathogens where it is clear that humoral immunity mediates protein. An example of this vaccine type is the hepatitis B surface antigen recombinant vaccine which has at least a 95% protective efficacy against hepatitis B.

### 5. DNA Plasmid Vaccine

The DNA plasmid-based vaccine is a novel approach that utilizes a mammalian expression vector which contains the gene of interest. This construct is then delivered by a number of different routes including intramuscular, intradermal or mucosal. It has been demonstrated that under the appropriate experimental conditions these constructs can be expressed and present the proteins generated to the immune system for the generation of specific immunity. This vaccine technology has been shown to function, in some aspects, similarly to a live attenuated vaccine preparation, as the proteins generated by these expression plasmids are processed as endogenous as well as exogenous proteins. Therefore, they are effective in generating helper and cytotoxic T cells as well as humoral immune responses. The potential advantages of this method, due to the ability to splice and modify specific genes, prevent the hazards of a live attenuated vaccine. This DNA vaccine technology is currently undergoing clinical evaluation.

## B. Routes of Vaccination

The routes of vaccination can be important as they affect the immunoglobulin isotype produced. Parenteral administration of vaccines (intradermal, subcutaneous or intramuscular) usually results in the production of IgG. Oral administration of vaccines produces IgA from the mucosal-associated lymphoid tissue (MALT), which is obviously desirable if the pathogen enters by the mucosa.

Adjuvants are agents that enhance the immunogenicity of vaccines and have been shown to be necessary for some vaccines to induce appropriately protective immune responses. Adjuvants are thought to work by (1) concentrating the antigen at sites where lymphocytes are exposed to it (the depot effect) as well as by (2) stimulating the production of cytokines. The only adjuvants that are currently approved for use in humans are the alum-based compounds. Other types of adjuvant preparations, including the direct use of cytokines as adjuvants, are currently being evaluated. In general, vaccines continue to hold a critical role in preventative medicine. Vaccination is the only technology that has resulted in the elimination of a human disease, i.e. smallpox. There are currently efforts by some groups to dissuade the public (including babies and children) from being vaccinated based upon supposed but false information that vaccination has a high and unacceptable risk. It is obviously important, through continued education of the lay public, to stop this dangerous trend or else the progress made in the prevention of a number of devastating infectious diseases through vaccination will have been lost.

## XIII. REGULATION OF IMMUNE SYSTEM AND DEVELOPMENT OF TOLERANCE

Immunity is controlled ultimately by exposure to antigen. Various other characteristics such as the route as well as the type and quantity of antigen can also have significant effects on regulation. Genes in both the MHC and non-MHC loci can have a significant effect in controlling the extent of immune responsiveness by mainly determining the T and B cell repertoires. Antigen-presenting cells provide co-stimulatory factors which boost immune responsiveness. Certain genes control the antigenic determinants that we respond to, i.e. the immune response repertoire. The major ones are the members of the Ig superfamily of molecules, such as the BCR (B cell receptor) and the TCR (T cell receptor), as well as the products of the MHC locus. These molecules are extremely polymorphic, allowing each individual to be unique in terms of which antigen they can respond to. Different cells of the immune system also have an important role in controlling the immune response. Th1 cells differentiate from Th0 cells and secrete IFN γ and IL-2 which help in the development of cell mediated immunity through macrophage activation and the elimination of intracellular pathogens. Th2 cells are also derived from Th0 cells but secrete IL4, IL5 and IL10, which help in the development of antibody and antiparasite immunity and allergy. The development of Th1 versus Th2 cells depends upon the cytokine environment, the type of APC stimulated, and the nature and amount of antigen given.

### Tolerance and Immune Nonresponsiveness

There are two potential response scenarios when lymphocytes are stimulated with antigen, and they can be either activated to induce an immune response or be tolerized to nonresponsiveness. When the lymphocytes are tolerized the responding lymphocytes can either be killed (i.e. clonal deletion) or rendered unresponsive (clonal anergy). In the process of development of mature T and B cells, tolerance or unresponsiveness to self-antigens occurs in primary lymphoid organs such as thymus.

In the thymus, T cells that respond to self-MHC are selected for while those responding to other self-peptides are selected against. In addition, T and B cells can be tolerized outside of the immune system. This occurs more readily in neonates, depends on circumstances of antigen exposure, occurs when cells are stimulated suboptimally (i.e. in the absence of costimulation) or follows negative signals from the APCs.

## XIV.  IMMUNITY TO TUMORS

Malignancies represent a cellular breakdown in normal growth regulation. Usually changes occur in the surface antigens of malignant cells that can often be recognized by the immune system. In general, immune responses against antigenic structures on the surface of tumors can be utilized for several purposes: (a) the diagnosis of cancer, (b) prophylaxis against cancer as well as (c) anti-cancer therapy. The concept of immunotherapy deals with the prevention of most tumors through early destruction of abnormal cells by the host's immune system. There is evidence to suggest that immunosurveillance does occur. This includes the observations that many tumors contain lymphoid infiltrates, which may be indicative of a more favorable clinical course as well as the observation that tumors arise more frequently in immunocompromised individuals. In addition, some types of tumors are more frequent in the neonatal period when immunity either has not yet sufficiently developed or when it is starting to senesce. It has been argued that unique tumor-specific antigens exist that are expressed only on the surface of tumor cells. However, the only confirmed tumor-specific antigens are the tumor-specific transplantation antigens (TSTA). These are molecules (antigens) that result in the generation of immune responses after transplantation of virally infected cells. Therefore, viral-specific antigens from oncogenic tumor viruses can likely then be considered the only true tumor-specific antigens. Tumor associated antigens are those that are expressed at a much higher frequency on tumor cells than normal cells. Examples of tumor associated antigens would include carcinoembryonic antigen (CEA) as well as $\alpha$ fetoprotein (AFP) and prostate specific antigen (PSA). In terms of immune responses to tumors there is evidence that both humoral and cell mediated immunity (CMI) can contribute to the suppression of tumor growth as well as spread of tumors (metastasis). However, CMI and specifically cytotoxic T lymphocytes are thought to be the most important. This is due to the fact that tumor antigens can be thought of primarily as endogenous antigens and thus engaging MHC class I antigen processing and presentation methods.

Other cell mediated immune responses include natural killer (NK) cells, which kill without antibody, killer (K) cells, which mediate antibody dependent cellular cytotoxicity (ADCC), and activated macrophages. The BCG vaccine (bovine-Calmette-Guerin, a bovine mycobacterium) as well as immunomodulators such as the interferons and interleukins have been shown through studies to have some anti-cancer activity as well as clinical potential. Two other immunotherapeutic methods to note are the LAKs and TILs. The lymphocyte activated killer (LAKs) are lymphocytes that have been activated which are then infused into tumors with the hopes of mediating anti-cancer activity. The tumor infiltrating lymphocytes (TILs) are removed from tumor tissues, purified, treated with IL-2 and then infused back into cancer patients. None of these modalities has been shown to be unequivocally effective in human cancer patients. Humoral immunity may play a role, albeit likely less prominent and important than CMI, against tumor cells. For example, IgG and IgM may fix complement and kill tumors. Antibodies could also interfere with the adhesive properties between tumor cells that are necessary for proper tumor development. Likewise, antibodies could kill tumors through an

ADCC mechanism. Monoclonal antibodies against tumor antigens also have other utilities. They can be used, when tagged appropriately, to diagnostically image tumors. Likewise, they can be tagged with radionuclides or toxins that can both target and kill tumors. The concept and interest in cancer vaccines have waxed and waned over the years. Interest is currently resurging in this concept mainly due to the advent of DNA recombinant technology. Various preparations and technologies, including DNA vaccines, are currently being investigated in their potential efficacy against malignancies.

## XV. IMMUNITY TO INFECTIONS

### A. Immunity Against Bacteria

Bacteria can replicate either extracellularly or intracellularly. Various bacteria can contain a variety of immunologically active antigen, predominantly lipopolysaccharide (LPS). In innate immunity, antigens such as LPS can interact with serum factors as well as immune and other cells to cause an early inflammation and influx of complement, phagocytic cells as well as cytokines such as IL-12. Antibodies play an important role in the development of resistance to bacteria and mediate protective responses generated by a number of bacterial vaccines. They can typically bind to proteins, preventing the attachment and subsequent infection of cells by bacteria. In addition, antibodies can bind to and neutralize toxins. Typically CMI consisting of activated T cells and macrophages is of considerable importance in combating intracellular bacteria. These types of bacteria are eliminated through cytokine activation of the host cells or the killing of these cells by NK cells and cytotoxic T cells.

### B. Immunity Against Viruses

Interferon ($\alpha$, $\beta$ or $\gamma$) is produced by most cells of the body in response to a viral infection. These interferons have been shown to have a viral replicative inhibitory activity and to also activate immune responses by enhancing the activity of APCs as well as NK cells. In terms of adaptive immunity, antibodies made against viral specific proteins can prevent infection by binding to and neutralizing viral particles through the prevention of attachment of the virus to host target cells. Specific IgA can be important in preventing the infection by viruses that infection through the mucosal route. CD8$^+$ cytotoxic T cells are the major line of defense against virally infected cells. CD4$^+$ T cells are also involved in antiviral immunity through the MHC class II viral antigen pathway. Once activated, these cells produce cytokines such as interferon $\gamma$ and TNF $\alpha$ which can subsequently activate macrophages and other immune cells.

### C. Immunity Against Parasitic Infections

Parasitic infections can be caused by single-celled protozoa to multicellular metazoans or worms. Eosinophils are often associated with resistance to worms and, when combined with IgE and mast cells, provide unique mechanisms of host resistance. CD8$^+$ killer cells are the major arm of the adaptive immune system which is involved in controlling infection by parasites.

## XVI.  CYTOKINES

The complex interactions between cells that are involved in the immune response are mediated by a series of low molecular weight proteins with a range of molecular weights from 6000 to 60,000. These immunomodulatory agents have been designated cytokines. They can serve as direct effectors, messengers or other regulators of cells. They can be involved in the inflammatory process, cell growth and maturation as well as driving specific immunoglobulin class switching as well as cytotoxic T cell effector function. Initially it was thought that each individual cytokine mediated a separate and distinct function. It is now clear that they each can have separate and unrelated functions. In addition the functions can be overlapping and may be additive, synergistic or antagonistic. In order for a cell to respond to a cytokine it must express a specific receptor. There are several groups of cytokines that have been identified and characterized. The inflammatory cytokines include IL-1, IL-6 as well as tumor necrosis factor $\alpha$ (TNF-$\alpha$). IL-1 is also known as the endogenous pyrogen and mediates febrile conditions after various infections. IL-6 and TNF-$\alpha$ are mediators of the acute phase response and vascular shock, respectively. IL-2 (T cell growth factor) holds a central role in immunology and is arguably the most important cytokine. It mediates critical roles in activating B cells, helper T cells as well as cytotoxic T cells. The T helper cell type II (Th2) cytokines is important in driving humoral responses. Important members of the Th2 cytokine group are IL-4, IL-5 and IL-10 as well as IL-13, which has similar functions to IL-4. In addition, IL-10 has been shown the inhibit cell mediated immune responses. In addition, IL-4 and IL-5 have been shown to be important in mediating immunoglobulin isotype switching. Other cytokines are released from type I helper T cells. These cytokines, IL-12, IL-18 and interferon gamma (IFN-$\gamma$), stimulate cellular immune responses such as cytotoxic T cells responses and often, as well, inhibit humoral immune responses.

Chemokines can be considered to be types of cytokines. They are a relatively large group of small polypeptides that play a key role in chemotaxis and the regulation of leukocyte traffic. It has recently been determined that some of the chemokine receptors serve as the secondary receptor for HIV. Therefore the specific chemokine ligands are being studied as inhibitors of HIV, which may give some clinical utility.

## XVII.  DELETERIOUS EFFECTS OF IMMUNITY

Immunity can have a down side. Some immunopathologic reactions occur when there is a breakdown of the mechanisms that normally prevent the generation of immune responses against self-antigens. Other pathological manifestations can result from responses to antigens that function as allergens.

### A.  Hypersensitivity Reactions

These types of reactions can be thought of as exaggerated immune responses that can result in damage. Four basic types of hypersensitivity reactions have been described, the first three being mediated by antibody (Types I, II and III) and the fourth (Type IV) mediated by cellular immunity, i.e. the so-called delayed type hypersensitivity.

## 1. Type I Hypersensitivity

Type I reactions are the most common type of hypersensitivity and can be described as allergic conditions such as hay fever, urticaria and eczema as well as the life-threatening anaphylactic reactions. Both types are mediated by IgE stimulated degranulation of mast cells with subsequent release of inflammatory mediators such as histamine. Other chemicals such as prostaglandins or thromboxanes as well as serotonin also have a role in these reactions. Some of the clinical manifestations include urticaria (hives), eczema and hay fever. The most severe manifestation of a type I reaction is generalized anaphylaxis characterized by hypotensive shock and severe bronchoconstriction. A prime example of a type I hypersensitivity reaction is hypersensitivity to wasp venom, penicillin or other drugs. Often these reactions are to metabolic breakdown products of the drugs which function as haptenic compounds (small molecules that cannot generate an immune response unless bound to a larger molecule) which bind to various body proteins. Drug reactions can produce a wide range of symptoms including rashes as well as more generalized manifestations such as systemic anaphylaxis. Treatment of the type I hypersensitivity reactions involves inhibition of the action of the mediators as well as support of blood pressure to prevent shock. Corticosteroids, antihistamines or cromolyn sodium (prevents release of harmful mediators) can be administered. In cases of systemic anaphylaxis, epinephrine can be administered to modulate and maintain blood pressure.

## 2. Type II Hypersensitivity

Type II reactions are usually mediated through IgG or IgM interactions with complement. The reaction mediates a cytotoxicity by affecting (by a "bystander" mechanism) red blood cells, leukocytes as well as platelets. Examples of this type of hypersensitivity include a number of autoimmune diseases as well as blood transfusion reactions. These manifestations can include thrombocytopenia, leukopenia and immune hemolytic anemia.

## 3. Type III Hypersensitivity Reactions

Type III reactions are immune complex mediated, again involving complement. Examples include the Arthrus reaction and serum sickness. The Arthrus reaction is an inflammation that occurs with the deposition of immune complexes at a particular site. Serum sickness is a more generalized inflammation resulting from the deposition of immune complexes throughout the body and may be characterized by a wide array of symptoms.

## 4. Type IV Hypersensitivity Reactions

Type IV hypersensitivity is also known as delayed type hypersensitivity. This type of hypersensitivity is mediated by cellular immunity (i.e. T lymphocytes). The response to the offending antigen is delayed (i.e. starts in hours or days compared to immediately). The major examples of medically relevant type IV hypersensitivity reactions are:

a.  **Contact Hypersensitivity.**  With contact hypersensitivity adverse reactions are generated against materials such as chemicals or metals (i.e. nickel, plants such as poison ivy as well as other materials such as soaps and cosmetics). The offending antigen can often be identified through patch testing.

b.  **Tuberculin Type Hypersensitivity.**  This type of hypersensitivity can aid in the diagnosis of infectious diseases. The classic example of this type of hypersensitivity is the establishment of exposure to *Mycobacterium tuberculosis,* the causal agent of tuberculosis, through the intradermal injection of tuberculin. In this test the development of redness and induration with a peak occurring at 2–3 days indicates infection, at some point in time, with *M. tuberculosis.*

## B. Autoimmunity and Autoimmune Disease

Autoimmunity represents a pathologic situation in which the immune system reacts against autologous antigens resulting in damage to tissue. Autoimmunity represents a failure of normal control mechanisms of the immune system. It is, in effect, a loss of tolerance. It is thought that the most critical step in the development of an autoimmune disease is the activation of self-reactive helper T cells, i.e. Th1 and Th2 cells which can induce cell mediated or antibody mediated autoimmunity. However, it is clear that most autoimmune diseases are antibody mediated. There are several mechanisms that have been put forth to explain the generation of autoimmunity although none of these has been unequivocally been shown to be responsible. These mechanisms include molecular mimicry in which cross-reactive antigens from bacteria and viruses result in the triggering of auto-reactive T and B cells as well as alterations of normal proteins and the release of hidden (i.e. "sequestered") antigens. For a number of autoimmune diseases there appears to be a genetic predisposition with distinct HLA associations.

A number of autoimmune disorders, some of which are serious conditions with high mortality, have been described. Some of the notable autoimmune diseases are multiple sclerosis, chronic thyroiditis, thrombocytopenia, type I diabetes, myasthenia gravis, hyperthyroidism, systemic lupus erythematosus, rheumatoid arthritis and Goodpasture's syndrome as well as the collagen vascular diseases such as scleroderma and polymyositis–dermatomyositis.

### 1. Multiple Sclerosis (MS)

MS is characterized by autoactivated T cells and macrophages that cause a progressive demyelinaton of the white matter of the brain. It is theorized that this condition may be precipitated by a viral infection, specifically a retrovirus, although this has not been firmly established as the data putting forth this hypothesis is controversial.

### 2. Chronic Thyroiditis

An example of this disorder is Hashimoto's thyroiditis in which autoantibodies are made against thyroglobulin, resulting in fibrotic lesions in the thyroid gland.

### 3. Idiopathic Thrombocytopenia Purpura (ITP)

ITP is the result of the generation of autoantibodies against platelets. This results in the destruction of the platelets in the spleen or through complement mediated lysis.

### 4. Diabetes

In some forms of diabetes, autoantibodies are generated to insulin receptors, which results in interference with insulin binding and a resultant increase in insulin resistance.

### 5. Myasthenia Gravis

In myasthenia gravis autoantibodies are generated against the acetylcholine receptors of the neuromuscular junction resulting in extreme muscle weakness.

### 6. Grave's Disease

Grave's disease (hyperthyroidism) results from the generation of autoantibodies against thyrotropin receptors which bind to and mimic the action of thyrotropin and thus stimulate the thyroid to produce more thyroxin, which results in the manifestations of the disorder.

### 7. Systemic Lupus Erythematosus (SLE)

SLE is characterized by the development of autoantibodies against DNA as well as other components of the nucleus. These antibodies result in the development of immune complexes and lead to the activation of complement, causing tissue damage including vasculitis and arthritis as well as glomerulonephritis.

Corticosteroids are often used as a treatment.

### 8. Rheumatoid Arthritis (RA)

RA is characterized by the development of autoantibodies (of the IgM type) against IgG. These autoantibodies are called rheumatoid factor, and they mediate tissue damage through immune complexes that activate complement. Treatment can consist of corticosteroids, anti-cytokine therapy, as well as methotrexate among others.

### 9. Goodpasture's Syndrome (GS)

GS is characterized by the development of autoantibodies to the collagen component of the basement membrane of the lungs and kidneys. It typically affects young men, and there is an increased risk of development of the syndrome associated with the expression of HLA-DR2. Symptoms of this syndrome can be severe and life-threatening if not properly treated. The symptoms include proteinuria, hematuria and pulmonary hemorrhage.

### 10. Scleroderma

Scleroderma (progressive systemic sclerosis) is an autoimmune disorder of unknown etiology characterized by a pathologic deposition of collagen in the skin. Immunologically, there are autoantibodies against topoisomerase I (Scl-70). This disease can affect the skin as well as internal organ tissues, which greatly increases the severity of the disorder.

### 11. Polymyositis–Dermatomyositis

Polymyositis and dermatomyositis are inflammatory diseases of the muscle and skin. They are characterized by autoantibodies to aminoacyl-tRNA as well as to other nuclear antigens. Muscle damage in polymyositis appears to be due to a cellular immune response mediated through the action of CD8+ T cells. In contrast, the pathology from dermatomyositis appears to be due to humoral immunity mediated through the action of CD4+ T cells.

## XVIII. REACTIONS BETWEEN ANTIGEN AND ANTIBODY: DIAGNOSTIC UTILITY

### A. Diagnostic Tests

As indicated elsewhere in this chapter, the interaction between antibody and antigen is highly specific. This exquisite specificity can be monopolized for the development of various diagnostic tests as well as analytical techniques that can be used in the research laboratory.

Serologic tests (i.e. based on antibody–antigen interactions) have significant applications for the diagnosis of infectious diseases, particularly when the organisms are not possible or difficult to culture. It also has applications for the diagnosis of autoimmune diseases as well as for the determination of blood and HLA type.

#### 1. Agglutination Reaction

Agglutination refers to the combination and interactions between an antibody and a particulate antigen that results in a clumping reaction that is visibly measurable. When antigen and antibody are in equal amounts, a zone of equivalence occurs with a resultant maximal precipitation. If either of the situations of antigen or antibody excess occurs, the precipitation is usually considerably less.

#### 2. Precipitation

In precipitation reactions the antigen is in solution; in other ways it is very similar to an agglutination reaction. This reaction can be performed in either agar or solution. In addition, the method can be performed in an electric field in which it is referred to as immunoelectrophoresis.

#### 3. Radioimmunoassay (RIA) and Enzyme-Linked Immunosorbent Assay (ELISA)

RIAs are highly sensitive assays that are based on the principle of competition for specific antibody between a labeled (i.e. known) and non-labeled material. Based upon this competition assay the concentrations of the unknown substances can be determined through the use of a standard curve. ELISAs utilize the same immunoassay principles as the RIA except that no radiolabeled materials are utilized. The method can be used to quantitate antigens or antibodies in patient samples and is nearly as sensitive as the RIA. This method of immunoassay is utilized extensively for diagnostic purposes.

## 4. Complement Fixation

Often immune responses (i.e. immune complexes) can be detected by the ability of these complexes to "fix" and "consume" complement. This assay can be utilized to detect immune responses to a number of infectious agents, such as viruses and fungi. However, in the wake of the development of more sensitive enzyme-based assays the complement fixation assay is often used as a confirmatory test.

## 5. Fluorescent Activated Cell Sorting (FACS)

FACS is a rather sophisticated test that measures the numbers of types of "immunologically active" cells. The technique monopolizes detection of specific cell surface markers on cells (i.e. the so-called CD markers). Specific monoclonal antibodies to these markers are labeled with fluorescent dyes. These cells are then passed through a laser light beam, and the number of cells that fluoresce is quantitated by the fluorescent activated cell sorter.

## 6. Western Blot

The Western blot is another immunoassay that is often used as a confirmatory test for an ELISA. In this assay proteins are separated on the basis of molecular weight by polyacrylamide electrophoresis, and the proteins are then electrophoretically transferred to nitrocellulose and reacted with antibodies and substrate for detection. The Western blot also has considerable utility as a research technique in addition to its diagnostic potential.

# B. ABO System, Blood Typing and the Rh System

## 1. ABO System and Blood Typing

The ABO alloantigens system is the basis for blood typing and transfusion. The A and B antigens are carbohydrate molecules on the surface of red blood cells as well as other cells. The possible combination of these antigens on erythrocytes are A, B, AB and O (i.e. no A or B antigen). If a person is A it means that he or she expresses two genes of A (i.e. AA) and has only circulating anti-B antibodies in the plasma. If a person is B it means that he or she expresses two genes of B (i.e. BB) and has only circulating anti-A antibodies in the plasma. Those who are AB express both A and B antigens (i.e. are co-dominant) and have neither anti-A nor anti-B circulating antibodies. Those who do not express either A or B on their red blood cells are type O and have both anti-A and anti-B antibodies circulating in their plasma. That is, the plasma contains the antibody against the "absent" antigens. This forms the basis for both blood typing as well as transfusion compatibility or incompatibility. That is, if a person's blood is mixed with specific antiserum against antigen A and this results in agglutination, then the blood type is A only if agglutination does not occur when it is mixed with specific antiserum against B. Agglutination with anti-B antiserum only indicates blood type B while agglutination with both anti-A and anti-B sera indicates blood group AB. Analogously, transfusion of a type A individual with type B blood would result in an incompatibility and lysis of the recipients RBCs due to the presence of specific anti-A antibodies in the donor's blood. Based upon these observations and principles, type O blood (i.e. with no anti-A or anti-B antibodies) can be considered to be "universal donors" while individuals with AB blood can be considered to be "universal recipients."

## 2. The Rh System and Hemolytic Disease of the Newborn

Greater than 80% of individuals have RBCs that express the Rh (D) antigen (i.e. are Rh (D)$^+$). It has been observed that when an Rh (D)$^-$ woman has a Rh (D)$^+$ fetus exposure of the mother's circulation to Rh (D)$^+$ expressing RBCs from the baby at birth induce the development of maternal anti-Rh (D) antibodies. Subsequent Rh (D)$^+$ pregnancies will usually be adversely affected since the maternal antibodies against Rh (D) can cross the placenta, bind to the fetal RBCs and lyse them, resulting in the condition known as hemolytic disease of the newborn, i.e. erythroblastosis fetalis. This condition can often be prevented by the administration of a preparation called Rho-Gam (a high-titer antibody preparation against the Rh (D) antigen) to the mother at around 28 weeks of gestation and again at the time of birth. These antibodies then attach to the Rh (D)$^+$ RBCs and prevent the Rh (D) antigen from functioning as an antigen, thus preventing the generation of anti-Rh (D) antibodies. This regimen is quite effective in preventing the hemolytic disease of the newborn. ABO blood group incompatibility can also cause a form of hemolytic disease of the newborn, but this is usually considerably milder than that caused by Rh incompatibilities.

## XIX. PRIMARY AND SECONDARY IMMUNODEFICIENCIES

Immunodeficiencies can typically manifest themselves as a deficiency in cells, (i.e. B cells, T cells or phagocytes) or a deficiency in complement. The immunodeficiencies can be either primary (i.e. congenital) or secondary (i.e. acquired).

### A. Cell Deficiencies

#### 1. Bruton's Agammaglobulinemia (X-Linked Hypogammaglobulinemia)

Bruton's agammaglobulinemia is a major primary B cell immune deficiency that affects young boys. In this condition there is a virtual absence of B cells and extremely low levels of all of the immunoglobulin classes. Female carriers of the X-linked defect are asymptomatic. T cell immunity in these individuals is generally normal. These individuals generally have recurrent infections with pyogenic bacteria. In terms of treatment, the administration of pooled γ globulin can decrease the numbers of serious infections. The molecular defect responsible for this condition is a mutation in the tyrosine kinase gene.

#### 2. Other B Cell Immunodeficiencies

Other B cell immunodeficiencies affect selective immunoglobulins of which IgA deficiency is the most clinically relevant. These individuals have recurrent lung and sinus infections.

## B. T Cell Deficiencies

### 1. DiGeorge Syndrome

One of the major T cell immunodeficiencies is DiGeorge syndrome in which the thymus fails to develop properly with a resultant severe deficiency in T cells. These children are characterized by recurrent severe fungal, viral and protozoan infections in early life. In some cases a transplant of fetal thymus tissue may result in the reconstitution of T cell immunity.

### 2. Hyper-IgM Immunodeficiency Syndrome

In hyper-IgM syndrome, patients (i.e. boys, as it is an X-linked disorder) have high levels of circulating IgM but very little IgG, IGA or IgE. This immunodeficiency occurs in the face of having normal numbers of T and B cells. Although affecting the production of antibodies, the molecular basis for this immunodeficiency results from a mutation in the gene for the CD40 ligand on helper T cells. This defect prevents the critical interaction between the CD40 ligand on B cells and CD40 on B cells. This defect prevents B cells from class switching from IgM to other antibody classes. This results in a severe decrease in the levels of circulating IgG. Treatment involves the administration of pooled γ globulin in order to decrease the incidence of infections.

## C. Combined B and T Cell Deficiencies

### SCID

The most significant and serious combined B and T cell immunodeficiency is the severe combined immunodeficiency disease (SCID). In this condition, because of significant defects in both T and B cells, recurrent infections early in life occur from viruses, bacteria, and protozoa as well as fungi. SCID can be either X linked or autosomal. The condition can be caused by a number of different mechanisms, including defects in (a) the IL-2 receptor on T cells; (b) the tyrosine kinase gene controlling important signal transduction events in immune cells; (c) the RAG 1 and 2 proteins that code for recombinase enzymes that are important for the generation of mature immunoglobulin molecules as well as T cell receptors; and the (d) adenosine deaminase activity. The T and B cell deficiency can be so severe that the children need to be isolated and protected from microorganisms. In patients with SCID, the use of bone marrow transplantation can sometimes restore immunity.

## D. Complement Deficiency

Various deficiencies in the complement system can result in immune deficits with a significant increase in the number of infections. Examples of primary complement deficiencies include hereditary angioedema and paroxysmal nocturnal hemoglobulinemia. Deficiencies predominantly in the C3 component of complement are associated with enhanced susceptibility to bacterial infections and sepsis by pyogenic bacteria such as *Staphylococcus aureus*. Deficiencies in components C5, C6, C7 and C8 are associated with enhanced susceptibility to bacteria caused by organisms such as *Neisseria gonorrhea* and *Neisseria meningitides*. Individuals with deficiencies in C2 and C4 exhibit signs of autoimmune diseases resembling systemic lupus erythematosus.

## E. Phagocytic Deficiencies

Primary deficiencies in neutrophil function can significantly increase the susceptibility to infections. In chronic granulomatous disease (CGD) there is an increased susceptibility to infection by *Staphylococcus aureus,* enteric rods and other opportunistic pathogens. CGD is due to a deficiency in neutrophilic NADPH oxidase which inhibits the microbicidal activity of neutrophils. Other phagocytic deficiencies which increase susceptibility to infections include (a) Chédiak–Higashi syndrome resulting from a lysosome deficiency, (b) hyper-IgE syndrome resulting from a defect in the ability of helper T cells to produce interferon γ and (c) leukocyte adhesion deficiency (LAD) syndrome due to a defective lymphocyte function associated antigen-1 (LFA-1) which results in inadequate phagocytosis of bacteria.

## F. Acquired Secondary Deficiencies

### 1. Malnutrition

Malnutrition due to the lack of consumption of critical amino acids can result in both B cell as well as complement deficiencies.

### 2. Common Variable Hypogammaglobulinemia

Common variable hypogammaglobulinemia is another acquired B cell deficiency hypothesized to be caused by impairment in T cell signaling. This rare condition affects adolescents as well as young adults. The condition is characterized by an increase in the incidence of pyogenic infections.

### 3. Acquired T Cell Immunodeficiency

Acquired immune deficiency syndrome (AIDS) is the most important and severe acquired T cell immunodeficiency. This syndrome became apparent in the early 1980s with the appearance of pneumonia caused by *Pneumocystis carinii* among homosexual men, an infection that normally almost exclusively occurs in individuals who are immunocompromised. It was subsequently demonstrated that a retrovirus, designated the human immunodeficiency virus, was the causative agent for this disease. HIV infects predominantly $CD4^+$ helper T cells and ultimately kills them, resulting in a profound suppression of cell-based immunity. The suppression of cell mediated immunity greatly increases the incidence of opportunistic diseases and malignancies in infected individuals. A number of the proteins of HIV are highly immunogenic, principally the envelope glycoproteins gp120 and gp41, with the result being that significant antibody and cellular (specifically, cytotoxic T cell responses) immune responses are produced in response to infection. In fact, there is some evidence that the cytotoxic T cell responses may have a role in maintaining, at least for a time, the asymptomatic phase of HIV infection. However, eventually with time the immune responses decrease with continued loss of $CD4^+$ T cells with the subsequent development of frank AIDS. However, the recent use of combinations of anti-retroviral therapies has been effective in keeping HIV viral loads very low or undetectable for extended periods of time. It is unclear how long these types of anti-retroviral therapies will continue to work, given the considerable nature of HIV to rapidly mutate over time. It is accepted, however, that the only effective way of halting the ongoing AIDS pandemic is through the development of an effective vaccine.

# Medical Bacteriology 3

*William W. Yotis, PhD*

## I. STREPTOCOCCI

### A. Classification

Streptococci are Gram-positive cocci that form chains, are catalase negative and are facultative anaerobes, but some are strictly anaerobes. They comprise a heterogeneous group of bacteria that are ubiquitous in nature. The major classification of the genus is dependent on the type of hemolysis produced on blood agar plates. Thus they can be $\alpha$, $\beta$, or $\gamma$ hemolytic. $\alpha$-Hemolytic streptococci partially lyse red blood cells in blood agar plates, which causes a green color around the colonies. $\beta$-Hemolytic streptococci completely lyse red blood cells in blood agar plates, which forms a clear zone around the colonies. *Streptococcus pyogenes* and *S. agalactiae* are $\beta$ hemolytic. Streptococci are classified as $\gamma$ hemolytic when they cannot produce hemolysis on blood agar plates.

Streptococci are also classified on a chemical basis. Lancefied classified streptococci on the basis of a cell wall polysaccharide called C-carbohydrate. For example, the specific C-carbohydrate for group A streptococci is a branched polymer of L-rhamnose and *N*-acetylglucosamine. Groups A, B, C, and G are $\beta$-hemolytic streptococci.

### B. Transmission

Many streptococcal infections are caused by streptococci acquired from other individuals or from the patient's own flora. These microbes are harbored on the nasopharyngeal mucosal membranes and on the skin of certain persons. Streptococci may be spread by airborne droplets and by contact.

### C. Pathogenesis of Group A Streptococci

The only species belonging to Group A is *S. pyogenes*. This organism produces many exotoxins and enzymes which play a role in infection: **(1) Pyrogenic exotoxins A, B and C, previously called erythrogenic toxins or scarlet fever toxins**—when small amounts of pyrogenic toxins are injected intradermally, they cause local erythema in persons susceptible to scarlet fever but not in immune individuals. This skin test is known as the Dick test. **(2) Streptolysin O** is oxygen labile, and cytotoxic for leukocytes, tissue cells and platelets. Antibodies against streptolysin O are formed during infection and are the basis for the antistreptolysin O test (ASO). **(3) Streptolysin S** is nonantigenic, oxygen stable and responsible for surface hemolysis around colonies of Group A streptococci. **(4) M-protein** occurs in more than 80 antigenic types. M-protein plays a key role for the establishment of Group A streptococcal infection, because it protects streptococci against phagocytosis. Strains of group A streptococci that do not produce M-protein are avirulent. **(5) Streptokinase**— This enzyme digests fibrin clots. **(6) Hyaluronidase** solubilizes hyaluronic acid of mammalian connective tissue. **(7) Deoxyribonuclease** depolymerizes DNA in exudates. Streptokinase, hyaluronidase and deoxyribonuclease may play a role in the spreading of streptococci in tissues.

## D. Diseases Caused by Group A Streptococci

### 1. Pharyngitis

It is associated with fever, chills, sometimes vomiting, erythema, purulent exudate and enlarged cervical lymph nodes. Pharyngitis due to *S. pyogenes* has to be differentiated from pharyngitis caused by adenoviral infection, diphtheria, infection caused by influenza virus, coxsackie virus, mycoplasmas, *Neisseria gonorrhoeae,* and human immunodeficiency virus.

### 2. Scarlet Fever

It consists of pharyngitis and a rash caused by erythrogenic toxins. The rash features small papules that give the skin a sandpaper-like appearance. There are also enlarged papillae on the tongue which is called "strawberry tongue." It should be noted that the production of erythrogenic toxins is controlled by a lysogenic phage.

### 3. Skin Infections: Impetigo, Cellulitis With or Without Erysipelas, Wound Infections, and Necrotizing Fasciitis (Gangrene)

a. **Impetigo** begins as red papules which change into vesicular and pustular lesions. These painless lesions coalesce to form honeycomb-like crusts. Impetigo caused by *Staphylococcus aureus* produces similar skin lesions.

b. **Cellulitis** is defined as an infection which involves the skin and subcutaneous tissues. Cellulitis with erysipelas shows bright red areas over the malar area of the face and the bridge of the nose. Superficial bullae may also form. Cellulitis caused by *S. aureus* produces similar lesions. As was the case with impetigo, the patient is only mildly ill.

c. **Necrotizing fasciitis (streptococcal gangrene)** is a severe disease that involves the fascia covering a muscle of the trunk or of an extremity. It features severe pain, fever, chills and erythema, and in hours the skin changes to dusky erythema and edema, there is marked tenderness, necrosis and inflammatory fluid.

### 4. Bacteremia, Puerpural Sepsis, and Toxic Shock-Like Syndrome

Bacteremia rarely occurs with uncomplicated pharyngitis, it may occasionally follow cellulitis, but it is common with necrotizing fasciitis.

When it occurs it can lead to pneumonia, endocarditis, meningitis, peritonitis, and osteomyelitis. Necrotizing fasciitis and cellulitis have been associated with toxic shock-like syndrome. This disease is usually linked to group A streptococci which produce pyrogenic exotoxins A, B, or C, and it causes fever, hypotension, respiratory distress or failure and renal damage. *S. aureus* causes the same disease with the only exception that patients with staphylococcal toxic shock syndrome are not bacteremic.

5. **Nonsuppurative Complications of Pyogenic Infections: Acute Rheumatic Fever (ARF) and Acute Glomerulonephritis (AGN)**

   a. **Acute Rheumatic Fever.** Up to 3% of patients who fail to receive effective antibiotic therapy for group A streptococcal pharyngitis may develop ARF 2–3 weeks after infection. The five major signs of ARF are carditis, migratory polyarthritis, chorea, subcutaneous nodules and erythema marginatum. ARF is due to cross reactivity between streptococcal M proteins and antigens of heart or joint tissue.

   b. **Acute Glomerulonephritis.** Few patients develop the classic picture of full-blown nephritic syndrome with acute oliguric kidney failure but most show periorbital and ankle edema, hypertension, and a urinary sediment with red blood cells, red cell casts, leukocytes and in few instances protein. AGN may occur 1–2 weeks after improper antibiotic treatment of pharyngitis or skin group A streptococcal infection, and it is associated with certain strains of *S. pyogenes* which possess M protein type 1, 2, 4, 12, 18, 25, 49, 55, 60 or 65. Type 49 is most frequently involved. AGN is thought to be caused by the deposition of immune antigen–antibody complexes on the glomerular basement membrane. Most patients recover completely from AGN.

## E. Diseases Caused by Pyogenic Streptococci Other Than Group A

### 1. Group B Streptococci

The representative species of group B streptococci is *Streptococcus agalactiae,* which is part of the normal oral and vaginal flora of women. It can be differentiated from *S. pyogenes* by its resistance to bacitracin and by its ability to hydrolyze sodium hippurate; it can also be differentiated with group B antiserum. It is the causative agent of neonatal meningitis, pneumonia and septicemia.

### 2. Group D Streptococci

This group includes the enterococci *Enterococcus faecalis* and *E. faecium* as well as the nonenterococci *Streptococcus bovis* and *S. canis.* Group D streptococci are resistant to bacitracin, grow in 40% bile, or pH 9.6. Enterococci grow in 6.5% NaCl, but not the nonenterococci. Group D streptococci are associated with endocarditis, intra-abdominal and urinary tract infections. Gastrointestinal and urinary tract surgery or indwelling catheters predispose to group D streptococcal infection, which can be a mixed infection. Enterococci are inhibited but not not killed by penicillin unless an aminoglycoside is added for synergy.

### 3. Viridans Group of Streptococci

These streptococci cannot be classified on the basis of the Lancefied's group-specific carbohydrates. Representative species include *Streptococcus mutans, S. mitis, S. intermedius* and the anaerobic bacterium *Peptostreptococcus magnus.* These organisms colonize the upper respiratory tract and are α hemolytic. *S. mutans* is the major cause of dental caries. The other organisms are associated with subacute infectious endocarditis, intra-abdominal infections, brain or liver abscesses, pneumonia and sinusitis.

## F. Laboratory Diagnosis

Group A streptococci are identified with specific group A antisera, pronounced β-hemolytic activity, susceptibility to bacitracin (0.04 unit) and inability to form catalase. The other groups are identified by their special features, which have been described previously.

## G. Treatment and Prevention

Group A streptococci are generally susceptible to penicillin G. For individuals allergic to penicillin G, erythromycin or azithromycin may be used. Immediate antibiotic treatment of suppurative group A infections usually prevents the development of acute poststreptococcal glomerulonephritis and acute rheumatic fever. Group B streptococcal infections may be treated with penicillin G and an aminoglycoside. The majority of viridans streptococci may be treated with extended use of penicillin G. However, many enterococci have developed resistance to penicillin, aminoglycosides and vancomycin. They present therapeutic problems, and linezolid has been approved for the treatment of vancomycin resistant enterococci.

## H. *Streptococcus pneumoniae*

### 1. Characterization

*S. pneumoniae* is a Gram-positive, lancet-shaped, encapsulated, α-hemolytic diplococcus. This organism is differentiated from other streptococci or staphylococci by its ability to ferment inulin, its sensitivity to optochin (ethyl hydrocuprein) and its sensitivity to bile. The pneumococcal capsule is composed of polysaccharides, of which there are 90 known distinct types. Addition of specific capsular antibody causes pneumococcal capsules to enlarge due to water absorption. This is known as the Quellung reaction.

### 2. Transmission

Humans constitute the only reservoir of infection for *S. pneumoniae.* This organism can be found in the nasopharynx of many healthy individuals. Thus the source of infection is endogenous, and pneumococci can also be transmitted by infected respiratory droplets.

### 3. Pathogenesis

The key virulence factor of *S. pneumoniae* is its capsule which inhibits phagocytosis. Non-encapsulated pneumococci are avirulent, and antibody to the capsule of a given type of polysaccharide provides immunity against infection of that antigenic type.

### 4. Diseases Caused by *S. pneumoniae*

a. **Lobar Pneumonia.** This disease is associated with sudden fever, chills, productive cough with red or brown sputum, pleuritic pain and possible consolidation of the lungs. The common predisposing conditions for pneumonia are splenectomy, which interferes with the proper clearance of pneumococcal bacteremia, defective antibody formation, defective complement function, alcoholism or cerebral impairment that may repress the cough reflex and prior viral infection. Lobar pneumonia is rarely a primary infection.

### b. Pneumococcal Meningitis

*S. pneumoniae* can reach the meninges following bacteremia and as an extension of otitis media or sinusitis. The classical symptoms of meningitis are sudden onset of fever, headache and stiffness or pain in the neck. If the infection is not treated with suitable antibiotics, patients may develop confusion, lethargy and shock, which can be lethal. *Haemophilus influenzae* is the most common cause of meningitis in newborns, but because of *H. influenzae* type b vaccination, *S. pneumoniae* now causes the majority of cases of meningitis in young children and infants. Also, with the exception of outbreaks of meningococcal meningitis, *S. pneumoniae* is the most common cause of meningitis in adults.

## 5. Laboratory Diagnosis

Laboratory diagnosis depends on the demonstration of lancet-shaped Gram-positive, encapsulated diplococci in rusty-looking sputum. Proper Gram stains of a sputum that has not been contaminated by oral bacteria show many diplococci, large numbers of polymorphonuclear cells and are free of epithelial cells. Cultivation of the etiological agent on blood agar must show α-hemolytic colonies which contain bacterial cells that are sensitive to optochin, are lysed by bile salts and can be typed by specific pneumococcal antisera.

## 6. Treatment and Prevention

The majority of strains of *S. pneumoniae* are sensitive to penicillin G or other β-lactam antibiotics. However, about one-fourth of pneumococcal strains are resistant to β-lactam antibiotics due to changes to penicillin-binding proteins. An extremely small number of pneumococcal strains are resistant to vancomycin, and thus vancomycin is the drug of choice for strains of *S. pneumoniae* that are resistant to β-lactam antibiotics.

Prevention of pneumococcal disease rests on a vaccine (pneumovax) composed of polysaccharides of the most common serotypes. This vaccine is recommended for immunocompromised persons, splenectomized individuals or persons older than 65. Pneumococcal polysaccharides of the most common seven types coupled to diphtheria toxoid can also be used to prevent meningitis and otitis media in young children.

# II. STAPHYLOCOCCI

## A. Characterization

There are approximately 12 species of staphylococci that may colonize the human body and thus be part of the normal flora. From the medical point of view, *Staphylococcus aureus* is the most important. Other medically important staphylococci are *S. epidermidis* and *S. saprophyticus*. Staphylococci are Gram-positive cocci that are arranged in clusters. They are catalase-positive, facultative anaerobic microbes. The primary feature that distinguishes *S. aureus* from other species of staphylococci is the production of coagulase. The name *aureus* is suggested by the golden color that develops when it grows on nutrient agar plates. On sheep blood agar plates, *S. aureus* usually produces β hemolysis. *S. epidermidis* forms white colonies on nutrient agar. *S. epidermitis* and *S. saprophyticus* are non-hemolytic. *S. epidermidis* causes urinary tract infections primarily in old age. Subacute bacterial endocarditis may occur in at least 2 months after heart surgery or after diagnostic invasive procedures and dental work. *S. saprophyticus* causes urinary tract infections in adolescent females.

## B. Transmission of *S. aureus*

*S. aureus* is ubiquitous in the environment. It can grow at 6–45°C, and it can be isolated from the external nares of about 30% of healthy individuals. Other areas that *S. aureus* colonizes are the axilla and the perineal regions. Health-care personnel are very prone to *S. aureus* colonization. Intravenous drug users and patients on hemolysis also have higher carrier rates of *S. aureus* than the general population.

*S. aureus* spreads from person to person usually by hand contact. On rare occasions it can be transmitted by aerosols from patients with staphylococcal pneumonia.

## C. Pathogenesis

The mechanism by which *S. aureus* produces disease is multifactorial, involving toxins, enzymes and cellular components.

1. **Enterotoxins A, B, C, D, E and H** cause acute gastrointestinal symptoms that are associated with *S. aureus* food poisoning. The enterotoxins are resistant to boiling and to the enzymes of the gastrointestinal tract.

2. **Exfoliatin or epidermolytic toxin** is the agent responsible for the production of staphylococcal scalded skin syndrome (Ritter's disease) in newborns and for the toxic epidermal necrolysis in older persons. This toxin is a proteolytic enzyme that separates the epidermis at the granular cell layer.

3. **Toxic shock syndrome toxin (TSST)** shares many biological features with the enterotoxins in that both are considered superantigens, that is, they can stimulate as many as 10% of the human T cells while normal antigens can only stimulate about one T cell per million T cells. This intense immune response leads to rapid production of interleukins 1 and 2, tumor necrosis factor and γ-interferon. TSST is the agent responsible for the production of the toxic shock syndrome.

4. **Alpha toxin** is an exotoxin that is lethal to many cells in low concentrations. It hemolyzes red blood cells, destroys platelets and causes skin necrosis.

5. **Leukocidin** is lethal to neutrophils by partially disrupting their membranes.

6. **Coagulase** converts fibrinogen to fibrin. In doing so it walls off the foci of infection, protecting staphylococci from host defense mechanisms and antibiotics. Also, coagulase-positive staphylococci grow well in normal human serum, while coagulase-negative staphylococci do not.

7. **Protein A** binds the Fc moiety of IgG 1 and 2 and thus hinders antibody mediated opsonization.

8. **Capsule.** The majority of strains of *S. aureus* isolated from clinical specimens possess polysaccharide capsules, which can interfere with phagocytosis.

## D. Diseases Caused by *S. aureus*

### 1. Toxigenic Diseases

a. **Staphylococcal Scalded Skin Syndrome.** This disease features periorbital and perioral erythema that spreads to the trunk and the extremities. Infants and children are irritable, have fever and are lethargic. These symptoms are followed by wrinkling and sloughing of the epidermis. This process may be repeated once. If the patient avoids hypovolemia, due to lethal electrolyte loss, or sepsis, recovery occurs in 1–2 weeks.

b. **Staphylococcal Toxic Shock Syndrome.** This disease is characterized by fever (102°F), diffuse macular rash, hypotension, vomiting, diarrhea, severe myalgias, renal and hepatic dysfunction as well as exfoliation of epidermis. This disease is caused by the toxic shock syndrome toxin.

c. **Staphylococcal Food Poisoning.** This poisoning occurs 1–6 hours following the ingestion of food containing preformed enterotoxin A, B, $C_1$, $C_2$, $C_3$, D, E or H. It features abrupt nausea, vomiting, diarrhea and abdominal pain. These symptoms subside between 5 and 24 hours.

### 2. Pyogenic, Suppurative Staphylococcal Infections

a. **Folliculitis.** It is a skin infection characterized by the formation of pimples, furuncles or carbuncles. A furuncle is a boil or superficial skin infection that develops in the hair follicle, sebaceous gland or sweat gland. Deep infection of interconnected follicles is called a carbuncle. Carbuncles are associated with intense inflammation of underlying tissues and may be complicated by bacteremia.

b. **Impetigo and Cellulitis.** *S. aureus* strains that produce exfoliatin toxin can cause bullous impetigo similar to that induced by *S. pyogenes*, which is also the major cause of cellulitis.

c. **Deep Infections Caused by *S. aureus*.** Hematogenous spread from a skin lesion can lead to bacteremia, endocarditis, pneumonia, meningitis, brain and spinal epidural abscesses, wound and kidney infections, osteomyelitis, septic arthritis and infection of any other tissue or organ. Foreign items such as intravenous catheters, sutures, heart valves and invasive diagnostic procedures constitute significant predisposing factors for staphylococcal infection.

## E. Laboratory Diagnosis

Observation of Gram stains of infected material reveals Gram-positive cocci in clusters with many neutrophils. *S. aureus* is coagulase and catalase positive, is β hemolytic, ferments mannitol anaerobically, tends to produce yellow colonies and grows well in media containing 7.5% NaCl.

*S. epidermidis* and *S. saprophyticus* are catalase positive, coagulase negative and do not ferment mannitol anaerobically. *S. epidermidis* is sensitive to novobiocin, while *S. saprophyticus* is resistant to novobiocin.

To trace the source of staphylococcal infection, staphylococci can be tracked by bacteriophage typing. Diagnosis of staphylococcal intoxications rests on the detection of the specific toxin responsible for the production of a given intoxication and on the clinical findings.

## F. Treatment and Prevention

Treatment of staphylococcal diseases requires the isolation of the etiological agent and the performance of antibiotic sensitivity tests because of the widespread resistance of staphylococci to antibiotics. Localized infections require oral antibiotics for approximately 10 days. Disseminated infections require parenteral antibiotic treatment for 4–6 weeks along with drainage of abscesses and removal of foreign bodies (catheters, etc.) when possible. Toxic shock syndrome, if it is severe, requires intravenous fluids and evaluation of blood pressure. Food poisoning is self-limiting. There are no vaccines available for the prevention of staphylococcal infections.

## III. GRAM-POSITIVE AEROBIC SPORE-FORMING BACILLI

### A. *Bacillus anthracis*

#### 1. Characterization

*B. anthracis* is a large (4–10 µm), Gram-positive, aerobic, spore-forming, encapsulated bacillus. It forms spores *in vitro* but not *in vivo*. Its capsule is unique in that it is composed of D-glutamic acid instead of polysaccharides. When observed under the microscope the organisms display a boxcar-like appearance. *B. anthracis* is a nonmotile rod.

#### 2. Transmission

Spores of *B. anthracis* can survive in soil for many years. The carcasses of animals dying from anthrax contaminate soil, air and water. Humans are accidental hosts, and anthrax is usually acquired when spores enter abrasions on the skin or when they are inhaled.

#### 3. Pathogenesis

The virulence of *B. anthracis* is a result of exotoxin production and the presence of an antiphagocytic capsule. The plasmid encoded exotoxin is composed of three proteins, called protective antigen (PA), edema factor (EF) and lethal factor (LF). By themselves these three proteins are inactive. However, when they are combined, they are very active biologically. PA and EF interfere with the phagocytosis and the oxidative burst of neutrophilic leukocytes. PA and LF can cause death within 1 hour of administration. PA binds to cell surface receptors and acts as a membrane channel, allowing LF and EF access to the host cell cytoplasm. EF is a calmodulin dependent adenyl cyclase and is believed to produce edema by increasing the levels of cAMP. LF induces influx of calcium and inhibits host cell macromolecular synthesis.

### 4. Disease Caused by *B. anthracis*

This organism causes anthrax which presents in three forms: cutaneous, which accounts for approximately 95% of cases; inhalational, the traditional woolsorter's disease, which is less common; and gastrointestinal, which is rare. However, all forms can lead to bacteremia, sepsis, meningitis and death. The incubation period of cutaneous anthrax lasts from 2 to 7 days. A patient with cutaneous anthrax presents with a pruritic macule or papule that enlarges into a round ulcer by the second day; 1–2 mm vesicles that discharge clear or sanguinous fluid might then appear. Purulent drainage usually does not accompany this lesion. This is followed by the development of a painless, depressed, black-colored eschar. The systemic symptoms include fever, chills, headaches and regional lymphadenopathy. If not treated early, dissemination of the disease can occur and does so in about 10% of cases, resulting in septicemia and meningitis. The mortality rate of untreated anthrax falls within a range of 5–20%.

### 5. Laboratory Diagnosis

Diagnosis may be made by soaking a sterile swab in the fluid of vesicular lesions. The Gram-stained fluid reveals the etiological agent under the microscope and on culture, unless the patient has been treated with antibiotics. For anthrax patients that have been treated with antibiotics, blood samples and skin biopsies of the lesion should be taken. Immunohistology of skin biopsies should reveal intact or fragmented *B. anthracis,* while polymerase chain reaction should reveal anthrax DNA in the patient's serum. Also, western blot testing of the patient's serum 1–2 weeks after the infection may reveal antibody response to the protective antigen (PA).

Differential diagnosis should include syphilitic chancre, erysipelas, glanders, plague and contagious pustular dermatitis caused by the pox-like orf virus.

### 6. Treatment and Prevention

High-dose intravenous penicillin and doxycycline are the antibacterial agents of choice, and these are given for 7–10 days. Ciprofloxacin is recommended for therapy of adults with inhalation anthrax.

Animals infected with anthrax must be buried intact or cremated. Face masks with biological filters that do not allow *B. anthracis* spores to enter the respiratory tract should be used by those at risk of exposure. Improved anthrax vaccines for humans are needed. The current vaccines composed of protective antigen or spores from attenuated strains of *B. anthracis* cause adverse reactions and provide incomplete protection.

## B. *Bacillus cereus*

### 1. Characterization

This organism is a Gram-positive, spore-forming, aerobic, motile bacillus.

### 2. Transmission

The spores of this organism that are resistant to to heat, germinate in certain foods, such as rice, and produce enterotoxins, which when ingested cause food poisoning.

### 3. Pathogenesis

Two enterotoxins are produced by *B. cereus*. The first one resembles the staphylococcal enterotoxins and is a superantigen. The second one is biologically similar to *Vibrio* cholera enterotoxin, and thus it is involved in the ADP-ribosylation of G protein.

### 4. Diseases Caused by *B. cereus*

This organism causes two forms of illnesses. The first one features symptoms similar to those caused by the staphylococcal enterotoxins. The second illness is an infection rather than intoxication, and thus it has a long incubation period (about 18 hours), which is followed by bloody, watery diarrhea.

### 5. Laboratory Diagnosis

It is not usually performed.

### 6. Treatment

*B. cereus* produces a self-limiting illness that usually does not require specific treatment.

## IV. GRAM-POSITIVE ANAEROBIC SPORE-FORMING BACILLI

### A. *Clostridium tetani*

#### 1. Characterization

*C. tetani* is a motile, anaerobic Gram-positive bacillus with terminal spores that resemble a tennis racket or a drumstick.

#### 2. Transmission

*C. tetani* is widely distributed in soil. It enters the human body following skin laceration, trauma, drug abuse, frostbite, burns, childbirth, abortion and surgery, and in neonates after unsterile treatment of the umbilical cord stump.

#### 3. Pathogenesis

Tetanus results from the production of *C. tetani* exotoxin (tetanospasmin). Spore germination and production of tetanospasmin in wounds does not occur unless there is sufficient dead tissue at the wound to provide a very low oxidation–reduction potential for the growth of *C. tetani*. Following production it is transported to spinal cord. It then migrates across the synapse to presynaptic terminals, where it interferes with the release of inhibitory neurotransmitters glycine and γ-aminobutyric acid. Furthermore, in a manner similar to that of the botulinum toxin, tetanospasmin can inhibit neurotransmitter release at the neuromuscular junction and produce paralysis.

#### 4. Disease Production

*C. tetani* is the causative agent of tetanus. The incubation period is 3–14 days. This illness begins with increased tone in the masseter muscles, which is known as lockjaw or trismus. At the same time there is dysphagia or pain in the back, shoulder and neck. Then, contraction of the facial muscles causes a sneer called risus sardonicus, and contraction of the back muscles produces an arched back known as opisthotonos. Few patients develop generalized spasms, which can cause apnea, or laryngospasm, which can be lethal.

### 5. Diagnosis

Bacteriological methods are of little value for the diagnosis of tetanus, which usually must be based on clinical findings alone. Electromyograms may show continuous discharge of motor units. Serum tetanus antitoxin levels of 0.01 unit/mL or higher are considered protective and render tetanus unlikely. Differential diagnosis for tetanus includes meningitis, encephalitis, rabies, hypocalcemic tetany and strychnine poisoning.

### 6. Treatment and Prevention

Human tetanus antitoxin is administered to neutralize circulating and free toxin in the wound, and with diazepam to control muscular spasms. Mechanical ventilation may also be required. Patients recovering from tetanus should be actively immunized with tetanus toxoid because the small amount of tetanospasmin produced during illness is not sufficient to provide immunity.

Tetanus can be effectively prevented by administration of the tetanus toxoid, which is usually given in childhood, but if the immunization status of the injured patient is not known toxoid is given in addition to antitoxin.

## B. *Clostridium botulinum*

### 1. Characterization

*C. botulinum* is a large, Gram-positive, anaerobic, spore-forming bacillus which produces the most potent exotoxin known. It requires a very low oxidation–reduction potential for growth and germination. The molecular basis for strict anaerobiasis is a lack of superoxide dismutase.

### 2. Transmission

*C. botulinum* resides in soil. Humans acquire botulism most frequently by the ingestion of preformed exotoxin in home canned foods that contain spores of *C. botulinum* and have not been properly sterilized. Exotoxin production is associated with spore germination.

### 3. Pathogenesis

Eight types of botulinum exotoxin are known: A, B, $C_1$, $C_2$, D, E, F and G. Types A, B and E cause human botulism. These exotoxins are polypeptides encoded by a lysogenic bacteriophage. They are neurotoxins acting at myoneural junctions to produce paralysis of cholinergic nerve fibers with subsequent suppression of acetylcholine release in peripheral nerves.

### 4. Disease Caused by *C. botulinum*

Botulism has an incubation period of several hours to a few days, depending on the concentration of ingested botulinum exotoxin.

Patients with botulism have dizziness, double vision, swallowing and speaking difficulties, dysphagia, muscular weakness, nausea, vomiting, respiratory paralysis and death in 20% of cases. Rare cases of botulism acquired by contamination of wounds by *C. botulinum* spores feature similar manifestations.

Illnesses that may be confused with botulism include diphtheria, poliomyelitis, Guillain-Barre syndrome, Lambert-Eaton syndrome, myasthenia gravis, hypermagnesemia, tick paralysis and intoxications from mushrooms, chemicals or medicines.

### 5. Diagnosis

The diagnosis of botulism is made by the demonstration of botulinum toxin in food, stool, blood or vomitus and by injecting mice and protecting them with botulinum toxin.

### 6. Treatment and Prevention

Treatment with trivalent antitoxin A, B and E should be initiated after testing for hypersensitivity to horse serum as soon as possible.

Prevention rests on proper sterilization of food and sufficient cooking to inactivate the heat labile botulinum exotoxins.

## C. *Clostridium perfringens*

### 1. Characterization

*C. perfringens* is an anaerobic, Gram-positive, encapsulated, nonmotile bacillus that forms large amounts of gas and subterminal spores.

### 2. Transmission

Spores of *C. perfringens* are widely distributed in soil, and vegetative cells are part of the normal flora of the gastrointestinal and female genital tracts. Gas gangrene (myonecrosis) is associated with deep trauma that follows motor vehicle accidents, gun shot wounds, septic abortion or other septic surgical procedures. *C. perfringens* food poisoning is the result of ingestion of food heavily contaminated with this microbe.

### 3. Pathogenesis

*C. perfringens* produces 12 exotoxins and enterotoxin. On the basis of production of four major exotoxins ($\alpha$, $\beta$, $\epsilon$ and $\iota$) the microbe is divided into types A, B, C, D and E. The $\alpha$ toxin is the most important. It is a phospholipase that destroys human cells by removing lecithin from human cells. Antibody to $\alpha$ toxin is protective against gas gangrene. The $\beta$, $\epsilon$ and $\iota$ toxins alter capillary permeability.

The enterotoxin of *C. perfringens* is heat labile, interferes with glucose transport and is associated with protein loss and damage of intestinal epithelium.

### 4. Disease Production by *C. perfringens*

a. **Gas Gangrene (Myonecrosis).** This infection has an incubation period of less than 3 days; it begins with localized pain at the site of the wound followed by local swelling, edema and hemorrhagic exudate. The destruction of traumatized tissue alone with hypotension and possible renal failure can then lead to shock and death.

b. **Food Poisoning.** This illness features abdominal pain with severe cramps and diarrhea for 1 day.

## 5. Diagnosis

Microscopic examination of the Gram-stained wound exudate. In gas gangrene, such smears usually show an abundant, diverse bacterial flora with large Gram-positive bacilli predominating. Pus cells either are absent or are few and degenerate. Wound and pus emit a foul smelling odor and may be frothy due to gas production. X-rays of wounds may reveal gas formation in tissues. Frozen-section biopsy can establish the diagnosis of gas gangrene.

Diagnostic assays for *C. perfringens* enterotoxin are not commercially available, and thus laboratory diagnosis for food poisoning caused by *C. perfringens* is not performed.

## 6. Treatment and Prevention

Debridement of necrotic tissue, penicillin G alone or combined with clindamycin.

## D. *Clostridium difficile*

### 1. Characterization

Slender, motile, Gram-positive, anaerobic, spore-forming bacillus.

### 2. Transmission

It is part of the normal flora. Antibiotic administration for the treatment of infections caused by other enteric bacteria allows overgrowth of *C. difficile.*

### 3. Pathogenesis

Toxin-mediated damage to intestinal wall. *C. difficile* produces exotoxins A and B. Exotoxin A is inflammatory, enhances fluid secretion and causes leakage of albumin from venules. Exotoxin B causes damage and exfoliation of superficial epithelial cells.

### 4. Disease Production

*C. difficile* is the etiological agent of antibiotic-associated pseudomembranous colitis. This illness causes voluminous, watery, diarrhea that is devoid of blood or mucus.

### 5. Laboratory Diagnosis

Detection of exotoxins A and B in the feces of patients with pseudomembranous colitis.

### 6. Treatment and Prevention

Administration of vancomycin or metronidazole. Prevention depends on cautious use of antibiotics and maintenance of the proper ecological balance between the normal intestinal flora.

# V. GRAM-POSITIVE AEROBIC BACILLI

## A. *Corynebacterium diphtheriae*

### 1. Characterization

*C. diphtheriae* is a Gram-positive, aerobic, bacillus that does not form spores, flagella or capsules. In Gram stain smears it appears club-shaped, and it is arranged in palisades or in the form of Chinese letters. Cultivation on the selective medium *tellurite agar* produces gray to black colonies. It grows luxuriantly on inspissated serum plates (Loeffler's medium).

### 2. Transmission

Humans constitute the reservoir of infection for *C. diphtheriae*. Transmission occurs by aerosols expelled from diphtheria patients and to a lesser extent by individuals who have recovered from diphtheria (carriers). Transmission by fomites is not common.

### 3. Pathogenesis

Diphtheria is caused by a potent polypeptide exotoxin that produces almost all the histopathology of classical diphtheria, that is, hemorrhage and necrosis within many different tissues. Only those strains of *C. diphtheriae* that are lysogenic for bacteriophage β produce diphtheria exotoxin. Nontoxigenic strains can be made toxigenic by exposure to bacteriophage β (lysogenic conversion). Detoxification of exotoxin can be achieved by treatment with formaldehyde, which converts the exotoxin to toxoid. The toxoid is used for immunization.

In vitro exotoxin production depends largely on the concentration of iron. It is composed of fragments A and B. Fragment B is responsible for the attachment of toxin to human cells and for the transport of fragment A through the membranes and the cytoplasm of human cells. Fragment A, once transported into human cells, inhibits protein synthesis, eventually killing the cells. Specifically, fragment A blocks protein synthesis by ADP-ribosylation of elongation factor 2 (EF-2).

### 4. Disease Production

The most common portal of entry for *C. diphtheria* is the upper respiratory tract, and the primary lesion of diphtheria is the throat membrane. The incubation period is 1–7 days. The outstanding symptom of diphtheria is the formation of an adherent, gray, thick membrane over the throat and the tonsils, referred to as diphtheritic pseudomembrane. This membrane forms as a result of the necrotic tissue action of *C. diphtheriae* exotoxin and consists of bacteria, necrotic epithelium, phagocytes, tissue exudate and fibrin. In the case of nasopharyngeal diphtheria, the membrane usually appears on the tonsils or posterior pharynx and spreads to the nasal passages or larynx. Laryngeal diphtheria is hazardous because of the danger of mechanical obstruction, and when this occurs intubation or tracheotomy is necessary to prevent suffocation. The systemic lesions of diphtheria are produced by the exotoxin circulating in the blood stream. The most common organs affected by the toxin are the heart, kidneys and the peripheral nerves.

### 5. Laboratory Diagnosis

Definitive diagnosis of diphtheria rests on the isolation of *C. diphtheriae* from lesions on tellurite agar and the production of exotoxin.

### 6. Treatment and Prevention

The primary treatment for diphtheria is administration of antitoxin, which should be given without delay. Because the antiserum used is derived from hyperimmunized horses, the usual preliminary skin test for sensitivity to horse serum proteins should be performed before the antitoxin is administered. Also a syringe containing epinephrine should be available for immediate use in the event of an anaphylactic reaction.

Penicillin or tetracycline should be given in combination with antitoxin to assist in the elimination of *C. diphtheriae* from the respiratory tract. It should be pointed out that antibiotics have no effect on the exotoxin. Tracheotomy is necessary when complete obstruction of the respiratory tract occurs.

Prevention of diphtheria depends on immunization of all children, who usually receive initial injections of toxoid at 2, 4 and 6 months of age and booster inoculations at 1 and 4–6 years of age. Diphtheria toxoid is commonly combined with tetanus toxoid and the pertussis vaccine in a single injection.

## B. *Listeria monocytogenes*

### 1. Characterization

*L. monocytogenes* is a Gram-positive bacillus that can grow aerobically or anaerobically at 1–45°C. It is arranged in L- and V-shaped formations resembling those found in corynebacteria. It is motile at 25°C, and it has a characteristic tumbling motion.

### 2. Transmission

*L. monocytogenes* can be encountered in soil, plants and animals. Contaminated dairy products, meat and vegetables are most frequently involved with the transmission of *L. monocytogenes*.

### 3. Pathogenesis

The ability of *L. monocytogenes* to survive and multiply within mononuclear cells has been attributed to the possession of a hemolysin known as listeriolysin O, a phospholipase C and a filament of actin called internalin which spreads the organism from cell to cell.

### 4. Disease Production

Serious infections can occur and are seen most commonly in neonates and immunocompromised individuals. Neonates acquire sepsis and meningitis from infected mothers. Organ transplant patients, persons with HIV infection and individuals receiving radiation or chemotherapy, whose the cellular immunity has been compromised, are good candidates for the development of sepsis and meningitis. The symptoms of meningitis are similar to those produced by group B streptococci. Foodborne transmission is important in listeriosis. An interesting feature of *L. monocytogenes* is its ability to grow at refrigerator temperatures.

*L. monocytogenes* may also survive pasteurization and cause gastroenteritis, which is characterized by abdominal cramps, fever and watery diarrhea.

### 5. Diagnosis

Isolation of *L. monocytogenes* from infected sites that are normally sterile, such as blood, spinal fluid or chorioamniotic fluid. Serotyping and DNA fingerprinting of strains associated with invasive or food infections.

### 6. Treatment and Prevention

Intravenous administration of ampicillin and an aminoglycoside for sepsis or meningitis. Patients allergic to penicillins should be treated with trimethoprim–sulfamethoxazole. Prevention rests on proper food sanitation and suitable prenatal medical care of pregnant women. Gastroenteritis is self-limiting and usually does not require treatment.

## VI. ACTINOMYCETES

### A. *Actinomyces israelii*

#### 1. Characterization

*A. israelii* is an anaerobic, Gram-positive, non-sporeforming, non-motile bacillus which forms long branching filaments. These filaments, in association with pus and calcium phosphate, form yellow masses in tissues called "sulfur granules."

#### 2. Transmission

*A. israelii* is part of the oral, intestinal and vaginal human flora. Thus the source of infection is endogenous, and there is no person-to-person transmission.

#### 3. Pathogenesis

It seems to be related to the ability of *A. israelii* to survive the host's inflammatory responses. This organism is an opportunistic microbe that does not produce any known virulence factor. Devitalized tissues, broken mucus membrane, presence of foreign bodies and immunosuppression promote the development of actinomycosis.

#### 4. Disease Production

Depending upon the site of initial infection, actinomycosis is classified as cervicofacial, thoracic or abdominal. The illness begins as a swelling or hard tumor with an uneven surface. As the disease progresses, abscesses develop with multiple draining sinuses and sulfur granules.

#### 5. Diagnosis

Detection of sulfur granules in abscesses with multiple draining sinuses and isolation of *A. israelii* from sulfur granules. Direct identification of *A. israelii* with the fluorescent antibody technique.

#### 6. Treatment and Prevention

Surgical drainage with prolonged penicillin or amoxicillin administration.

There is no vaccine available for the prevention of actinomycosis.

## B. *Nocardia asteroides*

### 1. Characterization

*N. asteroides* is an aerobic, Gram-positive, partially acid-fast, non-spore-forming, nonmotile bacillus that forms thin branching filaments.

### 2. Transmission

*N. asteroides* is found in soil, and thus infection occurs most frequently via the airborne route. However, it may enter the human body by implantation of *N. asteroides* into wounds, as is the case in actinomycetoma.

### 3. Pathogenesis

The mechanism by which *N. asteroides* causes disease has not been elucidated.

### 4. Disease Production

*N. asteroides* is an opportunistic germ that causes nocardiosis primarily in immunocompromised individuals. Nocardiosis starts as a pulmonary infection, which may later spread and form abscesses in the kidneys and brain. Puncture of the extremities and contamination of the wound with soil containing *N. asteroides* can lead to actinomycetoma. This infection features abscesses with multiple draining sinuses.

### 5. Diagnosis

Detection of Gram-positive, branching, thin filaments from multiple draining sinuses. Production of "breadcrumb" colonies on blood agar after 2–10 days of aerobic incubation. The organisms in these colonies are often partially acid fast.

### 6. Treatment and Prevention

Nocardiosis is frequently difficult to treat, but commonly sulfadiazine or sulfisoxazole is used. Abscesses in the brain, kidneys or extremities in addition to antibiotic administration may require aspiration, draining or excision.

There in no vaccine available for the prevention of nocardiosis.

## VII. MYCOBACTERIA

## A. *Mycobacterium tuberculosis*

### 1. Characterization

*M. tuberculosis* as well as other mycobacterial species of medical importance are aerobic, thin bacilli that cannot be decolorized by acid–alcohol and thus are acid-fast microbes. Acid-fastness is attributed to the presence of mycolic acid and other lipids of the mycobacterial cell wall. The high lipid content of the cell wall reduces the rate of entrance of nutrients in the mycobacterial cell, and as a consequence pathogenic mycobacteria require 1–8 weeks of cultivation to form colonies on the Lowenstein–Jensen medium that is used for their isolation.

### 2. Transmission

Patients with pulmonary tuberculosis spread *M. tuberculosis* to other persons by droplet nuclei, which are expelled by coughing, sneezing or speaking. In underdeveloped countries, unpasteurized milk from cows infected with *M. bovis* may transmit tuberculosis to humans.

### 3. Pathogenesis

*M. tuberculosis* does not produce exotoxin, endotoxin or any other virulence factor that explains clearly the mechanism of mycobacterial pathogenicity. The current belief is that the ability of *M. tuberculosis* to multiply within macrophages and kill them is the critical event in the pathogenesis of *M. tuberculosis*. The virulence of this organism has been associated with trehalose-dimycolate (cord factor) and the tuberculoproteins, which when combined with other cell wall waxes cause delayed hypersensitivity. The tissue damaging effect of delayed hypersensitivity is due to various cell wall lipids and cellular tuberculoproteins. Precipitation of tuberculoproteins from culture filtrates of *M. tuberculosis* yields a partially purified protein called purified protein derivative (PPD) which is used to test prior exposure to *M. tuberculosis*. This organism produces also what is known as repetitive protein that is thought to prevent the fusion of lysosome with the phagosome of phagocytic cells and thus escape its demise by the lysosomic digestive enzymes.

### 4. Disease Production

Tuberculosis is either pulmonary, or extrapulmonary. Prior to the emergence of human immunodeficiency virus infection, the majority of cases were pulmonary. Now, however, about 70% of tuberculosis cases are both pulmonary and extrapulmonary. Pulmonary tuberculosis can be classified as primary or postprimary (also called secondary, or reactivation, tuberculosis). Primary tuberculosis refers to infection in persons exposed to *M. tuberculosis* for the first time. The lung lesions formed are associated with hilar or paratracheal lymphadenopathy. In most cases primary lung lesions heal spontaneously and may leave a calcified node known as a Ghon nodule. In the lymph nodes the cell mediated immune response can be detected 4–6 weeks after infection by injecting intradermally PPD (purified protein derivative) of *M. tuberculosis*. The tuberculin skin test is read in 48–72 hours, and the extent of both induration and erythema is determined. A reaction of 10 mm or more is considered positive, and it means prior exposure to *M. tuberculosis* but not necessarily disease. The T cell immune response may stop the infection and prevent disease. This involves the production of nitric oxide and tumor necrosis factor (TNF-$\alpha$) by macrophages, and the synthesis of interferon gamma (INF-$\gamma$) by CD4$^+$ lymphocytes. Because HIV infected individuals tend to be deficient in CD4$^+$ lymphocytes, it is difficult to control the infection and disease caused by *M. tuberculosis* or by atypical mycobacteria (*M. kansasii*, *M. avium-intracellulare* complex).

Postprimary (secondary, reactivation) tuberculosis is an endogenous disease. It is the result of reactivation of a previous mycobacterial infection and a consequence of impairment of immune function by AIDS, corticosteroid treatment, chemotherapy or malnutrition. It may feature fever, night sweats, weakness, weight loss, cough with productive blood-stained sputum, hemoptysis, anemia, leukocytosis and caseous necrotic lesions which may spill to any organ, giving rise to extrapulmonary tuberculosis and seen now especially in patients with AIDS. In contrast to primary tuberculosis, calcified lesions of postprimary disease appear on the apex of lungs where the oxygen tension is high, favoring good growth of *M. tuberculosis*.

## 5. Diagnosis

Microscopic examination of acid-fast stains of expectorated sputum or of auramine–rhodamine stains provides presumptive diagnosis. Definitive diagnosis requires cultivation, isolation and identification by biochemical tests and DNA probes of *M. tuberculosis*. Other diagnostic procedures used include chest x-ray changes, positive skin test reactivity in the Mantoux PPD test and symptomatology. However, the clinical picture of tuberculosis shares some common features with coccidioidomycosis, histoplasmosis, blastomycosis, actinomycosis, nocardiosis, aspergillosis and other conditions.

## 6. Treatment and Prevention

Mycobacteria isolated from the Lowenstein–Jensen medium must be tested for susceptibility to common, primary antibiotics used, such as isoniazid, rifampin, ethambutol, streptomycin and pyrazinamide. Drug treatment is long (6–9 months) and requires bacteriological evaluation of the efficacy of antibiotic treatment and monitoring of antibiotic toxicity. Attempts have been made to prevent tuberculosis by use of isoniazid for people at risk of infection, such as children under 4 years of age who develop a positive tuberculin test, persons in close contact with tuberculosis patients and persons who are tuberculin positive and receive immunosuppressive drugs. Antibiotic prophylaxis is not effective against tuberculosis for entire communities, because the requirement that isoniazid be taken daily for 6–8 months cannot be met by the majority of people. BCG (bacillus-Calmette-Guerin) vaccination consists of attenuated live *M. bovis* cells. It is given only once and is recommended for underdeveloped countries where tuberculosis is very prevalent and for PPD-negative infants or children who cannot avoid prolonged and intimate exposure to patients with tuberculosis that is resistant to many antituberculosis drugs.

## B. Other Mycobacteria

They were disregarded earlier because they are not virulent for either guinea pigs or rabbits. Now their presence and simultaneous absence of *M. tuberculosis* in various human lesions has established them as human mycobacterial pathogens. They are called atypical mycobacteria because unlike *M. tuberculosis* they are not transmitted from person to person, their reservoirs are the soil, air and water, not the human body. They are divided into four groups, described below.

## 1. Photochromogens

These produce orange-yellow colonies only when they are grown with light. There are two photochromogens that are of medical importance: *M. kansasii and M. marinum. M. kansasii* causes chronic pulmonary disease indistinguishable from tuberculosis caused by *M. tuberculosis,* especially for individuals who have chronic bronchitis or pulmonary emphysema. Infected patients give a positive tuberculin test. The usual antituberculosis drugs are used for treatment.

*M. marinum* causes chronic granulomatous nodules and ulcers in the skin and subcutaneous tissues. Cases are associated with contaminated swimming pools. The natural reservoir of infection is fish. Infected patients give a positive tuberculin test when tested with PPD from *M. tuberculosis* or with PPD prepared from *M. marinum*. However, as is the case with *M. kansasii*, the mycobacterium which causes the infection gives a larger skin test reaction than the cross reacting organism. Minocycline or another tetracycline is used for treatment.

### 2. Scotochromogens

These mycobacteria produce colored colonies only when they are grown in the dark. *M. scrofulaceum* is a scotochromogen. This organism causes cervical adenitis (scrofula) in young children. Scrofula can also be caused by *M. tuberculosis*. Patients infected with *M. scrofulaceum* do not give a positive skin test with PPD from *M. tuberculosis*.

### 3. Nonchromogens

These mycobacteria do not produce colored colonies, regardless of whether they are grown in the presence of light or in the dark. *M. avium-intracellulare* complex is a nonchromogen. This organism causes chronic pulmonary disease which is indistinguishable from tuberculosis induced by *M. tuberculosis*. *M. avium-intracellulare* complex infections occur mainly in immunocompromised individuals such as AIDS patients, who are deficient in $CD4^+$ lymphocytes. Treatment consists of clarithromycin combined with rifabutin, ciprofloxacin, or ethambutol.

### 4. Rapid Growers

These mycobacterial organisms grow well at 22°C in 4–5 days. *M. fortuitum* and *M. chelonei* are rapidly growing mycobacteria. These usually saprophytic microbes may cause cutaneous infections, abscesses or corneal infections following trauma and pulmonary infections in patients with pre-existing lung disease. Immunosuppression, prosthetic hip joints and heart valves also constitute predisposing factors for infection by rapidly growing mycobacteria. Infected patients do not give a positive skin test with PPD prepared from *M. tuberculosis*.

## C. *Mycobacterium leprae*

### 1. Characterization

*M. leprae* is an acid-fast bacillus that cannot be cultivated in artificial media or in cell culture. It can be grown in armadillos or in the footpads of mice. It grows best at 30°C. Thus, normal body temperature protects deep viscera from *M. leprae*, which causes lesions in the skin and superficial nerves. This organism grows very slowly, with a generation time of about 2 weeks.

### 2. Transmission

Leprosy requires long and close contact with lepromatous patients who discharge *M. leprae* from their nasal secretions and from their skin lesions.

### 3. Pathogenesis

*M. leprae* does not produce any toxins and induces only slight inflammatory response. A surface lipid called phenolic glycolipid I may help protect *M. leprae* inside phagocytic cells by removing lethal superoxide anions and hydroxyl radicals. This may explain the ability of *M. leprae* to survive within phagocytic cells. The intensity of cell-mediated immune response also correlates well with the form of leprosy. Patients with tuberculoid leprosy display an intense cell mediated immune response and have few *M. leprae* bacilli in their tissue. Patients with lepromatous leprosy do not show any evidence of cellular immunity. Genetic constitution also seems to play a role in pathogenesis. For example, individuals with HLA-DR2 genes are likely to display the tuberculoid form of leprosy when infected, while persons with HLA-MT1 and HLA-DQ1 genes are likely to show the lepromatous form of leprosy.

### 4. Disease Production

Leprosy has an incubation of several years, and it presents itself in two main forms: *tuberculoid leprosy* and *lepromatous leprosy*. The tuberculoid form features blotchy red lesions with anaesthetic areas located on the face, trunk and extremities. These lesions are associated with an intense cell mediated immunity and pronounced delayed type allergic reactions. Few *M. leprae* cells can be found in the skin lesions when the disease becomes self-limited. However, tuberculoid leprosy can progress to lepromatous stage, which features a weak cell mediated immunity and many *M. leprae* cells in the affected areas with extensive skin involvement. Lepromatous patients lose their eyebrows, have thick nostrils, cheeks and ears, which give them what is known as a *leonine* (*lion-like*) *appearance*.

### 5. Diagnosis

Acid-fast or auramine–rhodamine staining of biopsies of skin lesions and nasal scrapings checks for anaesthetic lesions and appearance of granulomas. Injection of heat-killed *M. leprae* cells into the skin of patients with the tuberculoid form of leprosy may elicit a tuberculin-like reaction in 48 hours but not in patients with lepromatous leprosy (lepromin-skin test). Detection of antibody for the phenolic glycolipid I of *M. leprae* is thought to be 95% sensitive for the lepromatous leprosy and 30% sensitive for the tuberculoid form of the disease.

### 6. Treatment and Prevention

Dapsone (4, 4'-diaminodiphenylsulfone) combined with rifampin for the tuberculoid form of leprosy and dapsone, rifampin and clofazimine for lepromatous leprosy. Thalidomine for borderline lepromatous patients who have what is known as erythema nodosum leprosum.

Prevention rests on chemoprophylaxis with dapsone and isolation of persons with lepromatous leprosy.

## VIII. GRAM-NEGATIVE COCCI

### A. *Neisseria gonorrheae*

#### 1. Characterization

*N. gonorrheae* is a Gram-negative, oxidase-positive diplococcus that has flattened adjacent sides. It ferments glucose but not maltose. It is grown on the selective Thayer–Martin medium under 10% $CO_2$, but it is an aerobic organism. Strains of *N. gonorrheae* isolated from patients with gonorrhea contain pili. Avirulent strains of *N. gonorrheae* are non-piliated.

The outer membrane of gonococcus contains proteins I–III (OPAs) and a polysaccharide-like macromolecule known as lipooligosaccharide (LOS, not LPS).

### 2. Transmission

Humans constitute the only natural reservoir of infection for *N. gonorrheae*. Transmission of gonorrhea occurs by sexual intercourse or intimate contact. Infection of the conjunctiva of the newborn (ophthalmia neonatorum) is acquired by passage of babies through an infected birth canal.

### 3. Pathogenesis

Virulent strains of *N. gonorrheae* have pili that allow them to adhere to human columnar epithelial cells, and antibodies to a given antigenic type of pilus prevent infection. Unfortunately, pili undergo extensive antigenic and phase variation, which explains why the same strain of *N. gonorrheae* can cause repeated infections in the same individual. Pili may also inhibit phagocytosis by neutrophils. OPA II, like pili, serves as an adhesion. OPA I molecules combine to form outer membrane (porins) which allow hydrophilic molecules to pass through the gonococcal cell wall outer membrane. The lipooligosaccharide (LOS) stimulates the production of tumor necrosis factor, which in turn may cause inflammation and tissue damage. This tissue damage can be inhibited by specific antibody to tumor necrosis factor. Finally, evasion of the host immune defense has been attributed to antigenic variation of LOS. Gonococci produce various hydrolytic enzymes which have been associated with the virulence of *N. gonorrheae*. *IgA protease* hydrolyzes the secretory immunoglobulin IgA, which interferes with the attachment of gonococci to human columnar and transitional epithelium. Dissemination of gonococci in the human body depends not only on the virulence factors of *N. gonorrheae* but also upon the absence of certain complement components. For example, individuals deficient in complement components $C_6$ to $C_9$ are at risk of developing gonococcemia with purulent arthritis, myopericarditis, toxic hepatitis, endocarditis or meningitis.

### 4. Disease Production

In most instances the primary focus of infection is the urethral epithelium in the male and the endocervix epithelium in the female. *Urethritis* in males features painful urination and purulent urethral discharge 2–5 days after exposure. In the female, urethritis is associated with painful and frequent urination. Endocervical gonococcal infection features a yellow vaginal discharge, while infection of Bartholin's gland causes labial pain and swelling of the gland. Extension of urethritis or cervicitis may lead to pelvic inflammatory disease (PID), endomitritis and salpingitis, which can result in sterility or ectopic prepregnancy. Extension through the blood stream results in arthritis–dermatitis syndrome featuring pustules distributed on distal extremities plus asymmetrical arthralgias, tenosynovitis or arthritis involving knees, ankles, wrists and small joints of hands and feet. Rarely endocarditis and meningitis can occur.

*N. gonorrheae* may cause ophthalmia neonatorum in babies who pass through an infected birth canal and vulvovaginitis in young children who in few instances may acquire this infection from infected towels and linen.

*Chlamydia trachomatis,* which is the most common cause of pelvic inflammatory disease (PID), shares many clinical features found in gonococcal disease.

## 5. Diagnosis

Provisional diagnosis of gonococcal infection can be made by demonstrating many Gram-negative diplococci with flattened adjacent ends inside polymorphonuclear cells in Gram-stained smears of purulent discharges. Definitive diagnosis of gonococcal illness requires cultivation, isolation and identification of *N. gonorrheae.* Specimens from urethra, cervix, anus, rectum and pharynx that are usually contaminated with normal flora should be cultured on Thayer–Martin medium that contains antibiotics which selectively inhibit most other microorganisms. Specimens not likely to be contaminated, such as blood or synovial fluid, should be cultured on chocolate agar. All types of media should be incubated in 5–10% $CO_2$. Isolated colonies must be confirmed by oxidase tests, Gram staining, utilization of glucose but not maltose and, when necessary, nucleic acid probes. An enzyme-linked immunosorbent assay may also be used to detect gonococcal antigen in urethral or cervical secretions.

## 6. Treatment and Prevention

For uncomplicated infection of urethra, cervix, rectum or pharynx, ceftriaxone, cefoxime, ciprofloxacin, ofloxacin plus doxycycline for possible coinfection with *Chlamydia trachomatis.* Alternative regimens include spectinomycin, ceftizoxime and cefotaxime. For disseminated gonococcal infection, ceftriaxone.

Prevention of gonococcal disease rests on the use of condoms and proper antibiotic treatment of infected individuals plus their contacts. Ophthalmia neonatorum of the newborn can be prevented with an erythromycin ointment.

# B. *Neisseria meningitidis*

## 1. Characterization

*N. meningitidis* is in many respects similar to *N. gonorrheae.* Both organisms also die quickly once removed from the human body and thus require bedside cultures for isolation from clinical specimens. *N. meningitidis* can be conveniently differentiated from *N. gonorrheae* by its ability to ferment maltose and the possession of a very well defined capsule. Meningococci are divided into at least 13 serologic groups on the basis of the antigenic differences of the capsular polysaccharides. Groups A, B, C, 29E, W-135 and Y cause more than 99% of meningococcal infections. Serogroup A meningococci are primarily involved in epidemics.

## 2. Transmission

Like *N. gonorrheae, N. meningitidis* is strictly a human pathogen that resides in the nasopharynx. During nonepidemic periods the nasopharyngeal carriage is about 10%. *N. meningitidis* is transmitted by inhalation of infected airborne droplets and by direct or indirect oral contact.

## 3. Pathogenesis

The production of capsule, endotoxin (LPS) and IgA protease are the major virulence factors that involve in the pathogenesis of gonococcal disease. Capsules interfere with phagocytosis. Resistance to meningococci coincides with the presence of the antibody specific for an antigenic group of capsular polysaccharide. Endotoxin induces fever, hypotension, shock, inflammation, disseminated intravascular coagulation (DIC), tissue necrosis by stimulating the production of tumor necrosis factor, rashes and tissue ischemia, which are all signs of meningococcemia. The concentration of LPS in the plasma of patients with meningococcemia coincides with the severity of illness.

The incidence of meningitis in sub-Saharan Africa rises during dusty seasons, and this has been attributed to reduced production of IgA in the nasopharynx by dust. IgA protease intensifies this problem by degrading IgA and thus allowing gonococci to attach to human cells.

### 4. Disease Production

*N. meningitidis* produces most commonly meningitis, usually striking infants less than 1 year old. Meningitis has an incubation period of 1–3 days and is characterized by irritability, fever, vomiting and lethargy. Infants have a bulging anterior fontanelle, while older patients have a stiff neck and positive Kernig's and Brudzinski's signs. There is often a hemorrhagic skin rash with petechiae, indicating an associated meningococcemia. Invasion of the bloodstream may take the form of a fulminant meningococcemia known as the Waterhouse–Friderichsen syndrome. This illness is characterized by rapidly enlarging petechiae, tachycardia, hypotension, arthralgia, disseminated intravascular coagulation (DIC), adrenal insufficiency, shock, coma or death. Skin rashes, such as viral exanthems, rose spots of typhoid fever, Rocky Mountain spotted fever, endemic typhus, *Mycoplasma* disease, and vascular purpura, may be confused with those produced by *N. meningitidis*.

### 5. Diagnosis

The diagnosis of meningococcal disease is made as it was described for *N. gonorrheae*. *N. meningitidis* ferments maltose and glucose, while *N. gonorrheae* ferments glucose but not maltose.

### 6. Treatment and Prevention

The mortality rate of untreated meningococcal disease can be as high as 60%. Thus antibiotic therapy must be instituted with intravenous penicillin G or ampicillin, if the diagnosis is suspected, without awaiting confirmation. Prevention of meningococcal disease may be achieved by rifampin chemoprophylaxis and vaccination with capsular polysaccharide derived from group A, C, Y and W-135 strains. The capsular polysaccharide derived from group B strains is weakly antigenic, and thus vaccination with this polysaccharide is ineffective.

## IX. GRAM-NEGATIVE RODS CAUSING RESPIRATORY TRACT ILLNESS

### A. *Haemophilus influenzae*

#### 1. Characterization

*H. influenzae* is a minute, pleomorphic, facultative anaerobic, Gram-negative bacillus. When grown aerobically it requires nicotinamide adenine dianucleotide (factor V) and hemin (factor X). There are six antigenic types of *H. influenzae:* a, b, c, d, e and f. Antigenic typing is based on the composition of the capsular polysaccharides. The capsule of *H. influenzae* type b (Hib), which causes severe, invasive disease, is composed of ribosylribitol phosphate. Nontypable strains of *N. influenzae* do not possess capsules, are usually noninvasive and have been associated with sinusitis and otitis media in children.

## 2. Transmission

*H. influenzae* is strictly a human pathogen and is transmitted from person to person by airborne droplets or by contact with contaminated fomites.

## 3. Pathogenesis

The main virulence factor of Hib is its capsule, which inhibits phagocytosis. Immunization with the capsular polysaccharide ribosylribitol phosphate is now used to protect infants 2–6 months of age. The mechanism of pathogenesis for nontypable strains of *H. influenzae* has not been elucidated.

## 4. Disease Production by *H. influenzae* Type b

First, this organism causes a very important disease, which is meningitis. This severe illness produces headache, fever, drowsiness and stiff neck. Second, it can cause sinusitis and otitis media similar to that produced by *S. pneumoniae*. Third, in rare occasions, it can cause epiglotitis, which is a life-threatening illness because it can lead to obstruction of the upper respiratory tract.

Untypable strains of *H. influenzae* may cause pneumonia in individuals with chronic respiratory infections.

*H. influenzae* biogroup *aegyptius* can cause conjunctivitis and Brazilian purpuric fever (BPF) in children 3–96 months of age. BPF follows purulent conjunctivitis, with high fever, vomiting, abdominal pain, petechiae, purpura and peripheral necrosis, and it can lead to vascular collapse.

## 5. Diagnosis

Demonstration of Gram-negative coccobacilli in Gram stains of CSF obtained from patients with meningitis provides good evidence for Hib meningitis. Confirmation of Hib illness requires cultivation on chocolate agar and identification by fluorescent antibody staining, latex agglutination tests and detection of Hib capsular polysaccharide in CSF, blood or other clinical specimen.

## 6. Treatment and Prevention

Meningitis caused by Hib is first treated with ceftriaxone or cefotaxime for 1–2 weeks. Persons sensitive to these antibiotics may be treated with ampicillin and chloramphenicol. Dexamethasone may be used to reduce the incidence of possible neurologic sequelae, such as hearing loss, or delay in language development. Epiglotitis is a medical emergency and requires maintenance of an open airway.

Prevention rests on immunization of all children with Hib conjugate vaccine (composed of Hib capsular polysaccharide conjugated to diphtheria toxoid), which is administered at 2–15 months of age. Household contacts of patients with Hib illness may be protected with oral rifampin.

### B. *Bordetella pertussis*

#### 1. Characterization

*B. pertussis* is an aerobic, nonmotile, encapsulated, Gram-negative coccobacillus, but is sometimes pleomorphic, similar to *H. influenzae*. It is delicate and fastidious. It is usually grown on Bordet–Gengou agar, which is a rich growth medium containing blood. *B. pertussis* is the etiological agent of whooping cough, which is exclusively a human disease.

#### 2. Transmission

Whooping cough is acquired by inhalation of respiratory droplets produced by infected individuals.

#### 3. Pathogenesis

*B. pertussis* produces such virulence factors as the antiphagocytic capsule; the fimbriae, which allow the organism to adhere initially to ciliated cells; a filamentous hemagglutinin, which with another outer membrane protein called pertactin, can allow *B. pertussis* to adhere tightly to ciliated and other human cells; a tracheal cytotoxin, which induces ciliostasis; an antiphagocytic adenyl cyclase; and the pertussis toxin that transfers ADP-ribose to regulatory membrane G proteins of the human target cells that leads to the production of the lymphocytosis-promoting and the histamine sensitizing factors.

#### 4. Disease Production

Whooping cough is a non-invasive, very contagious disease that tends to affect newborns and infants. In its classic picture, three stages follow an incubation period of approximately 10 days. Thus, there is the catarrhal or prodromal stage of 1–2 weeks' duration, with symptoms similar to mild upper respiratory infection when the disease is most communicable. The paroxysmal stage then follows within 1–6 weeks. During this stage the sudden, forceful, repetitive cough occurs (paroxysmal cough). The characteristic whoop occurs in about 50% of cases, and it is caused by the sudden inspiration against a closed glottis when the paroxysmal cough ends. It may also be associated with anorexia, vomit aspiration and secondary infections, such as pneumonia with other microbes. Lymphocytosis occurs during both the catarrhal and paroxysmal stages of whooping cough. Rare complications such as encephalopathy and seizures have also been observed.

The paroxysmal stage of the disease subsides in several months, and the convalescent stage finally sets in.

#### 5. Diagnosis

Confirmation of whooping cough requires the isolation of *B. pertussis* from nasopharyngeal calcium alginate swabs. Identification of the causative agent can be made by agglutination with specific antiserum or by enzyme-linked immunosorbent assays. When the patient has received antibiotics, detection of *B. pertussis* DNA in nasopharyngeal specimens by the polymerase chain reaction can be used.

## 6. Treatment and Prevention

Treatment early during the prodromal stage with erythromycin will generally lessen the severity of the paroxysmal stage, but it will not prevent it. Furthermore, treatment before any symptoms appear may prevent an epidemic spread. Finally, treatment of contacts is important, and secondary infections should be treated with appropriate antibiotics.

Prevention of whooping cough requires immunization with whole heat killed *B. pertussis* cells or an acellular vaccine. The vaccine is combined with the diphtheria and tetanus toxoid, and it is administered at 2, 4, 8, 15–18 months and at 4–6 years of age. The key immunogen of the acellular vaccine is the inactivated pertussis toxin, which produces fewer adverse reactions than the cellular vaccine and induces strong antibody response in adults.

# C. *Legionella pneumophila*

## 1. Characterization

*L. pneumophila* is a thin, aerobic, faintly stained Gram-negative rod. It is usually grown on charcoal yeast extract agar that is supplemented with large amounts of cysteine which is an absolute requirement for growth of *L. pneumophila*.

## 2. Transmission

This microbe is found in water, and it enters the human body by aerosolization, aspiration and direct instillation into the lungs during respiratory tract manipulation. Aerosolization of *L. pneumophila* by humidifiers, ultrasonic mist machines, air conditioning units, showers and nebulizers have been implicated in the transmission of *L. pneumophila*.

## 3. Pathogenesis

The mechanism by which *L. pneumophila* produces disease is unclear, but survival within macrophages is important. It has been stated that once the bacterial cells have been phagocytosed they appear to inhibit the fusion of the phagosome with lysosome which usually results in the release of various antibacterial substances. Host predisposition such as immunosuppression and chronic lung disease facilitate illness by *L. pneumophila*.

## 4. Disease Production

Eighty to 90% of Legionnaire's disease (pneumonia) is caused by *Legionella pneumophila*; the remainder is due to *L. micdadei* or *L. bozemanii*. The symptoms vary from a mild flu-like illness to severe pneumonia with fever over 40.5°C, nonproductive cough, confusion, headache, chills, vomiting, nonbloody diarrhea, pulmonary infiltrates, hyponatremia and multisystem failure. These symptoms resemble those produced by *Chlamydia pneumoniae, Chlamydia psittaci, Mycoplasma pneumoniae, Coxiella burnetii* and various viruses. These microbes have their unique characteristics and thus differentiation is made on this basis.

**Pontiac fever** is another infection caused by *L. pneumophila*. This illness is characterized by malaise, fever, chills, fatigue and myalgias, but not pneumonia, and it lasts 1–2 days.

### 5. Diagnosis

Definitive diagnosis of *Legionella* illness depends on the isolation of the etiological agent on charcoal yeast extract agar. Direct fluorescent antibody tests performed on bronchoalveolar lavage fluids, pleural effusions or sputa and demonstration of a four-fold rise in antibody titer against *L. pneumophila* are also very useful.

### 6. Treatment and Prevention

Diseases caused by pathogenic legionella organisms are usually treated with erythromycin alone or in combination with refampin.

Prevention rests on disinfection of water supply by heat or the copper and silver ionization method.

## X. ANIMAL GRAM-NEGATIVE RODS CAUSING HUMAN DISEASE

### A. Brucellae

#### 1. Characterization

*Brucella abortus, Brucella melitensis* and *Brucella suis* are the three species of brucellae that are of medical importance. *B. abortus* infects cattle and man, requires 10% $CO_2$ for primary isolation, contains large amounts of antigen A and it is inhibited by the dye thionine. *B. melitensis* infects goats and man and contains large amounts of antigen M. *B. suis* infects swine and man, and it is inhibited by the dye basic fuchsin. These microbes are very small aerobic, nonmotile, nonencapsulated, non-spore-forming, Gram-negative, facultative intracellular bacilli. They are killed by pasteurization.

#### 2. Transmission

Individuals acquire brucellosis (undulant fever, Malta fever, Bang's disease) by ingestion of infected dairy products, by inhalation of infected particles and by contact with infected tissues of animals.

#### 3. Pathogenesis

The mechanism by which brucellae produce disease remains unknown. However, virulence has been associated with the ability of the microbes to survive intracellularly, especially in the bone marrow, liver and spleen. The endotoxin also appears to be involved. Erythritol is a growth stimulant and explains why animals with high levels of erythritol in their placenta abort while humans with low levels of erythritol in their placenta do not abort. Finally, hypersensitivity to *Brucella* antigens may explain the production of granulomatous lesions seen in various tissues.

#### 4. Disease Production

Brucellosis features diverse clinical symptoms depending on the severity and site of infection. The incubation period lasts 1–8 weeks, and the most common signs include fatigue, anorexia, headache, fever, chills, sore throat, dry cough, diaphoresis, constipation, weight loss, agitation and joint and low back pain. The symptoms occur because the organisms invade the entire reticuloendothelial system and often involve bones and joints, respiratory tract, gastrointestinal tract, genitourinary tract, central nervous system, heart, eyes and skin.

### 5. Diagnosis

Culture of blood taken during pyrexia, or biopsy material from lymph nodes, bone marrow, spleen or liver in 10% $CO_2$ for at least 6 weeks. Agglutination tests to show rise in antibody titer. Titer above 1:80 indicates past or present infection. Persons vaccinated with cholera vaccine may develop agglutinin titers to brucella; however, those titers are lower than those obtained for brucella. Blocking (univalent) antibodies, which are β-globulins, may produce negative agglutination tests in late brucellosis. Precipitin assays may alleviate this problem, however.

### 6. Treatment and Prevention

Doxycycline combined with streptomycin, gentamicin or netilmicin for 4 weeks, followed by doxycycline and rifampin for 4–8 weeks. Prolonged treatment is necessary because of the intracellular location of *Brucella*.

Prevention requires proper sanitary measures, pasteurization of dairy products, elimination of infected animals and vaccination of cattle, goats and swine with a live attenuated vaccine.

## B. *Francisella tularensis*

### 1. Characterization

*F. tularensis,* the causative agent of tularemia, is an encapsulated, aerobic, nonmotile, pleomorphic Gram-negative bacillus with bipolar staining that results in coccoid appearance. It requires cysteine in amounts exceeding those usually present in nutrient media, and it grows best on cysteine glucose blood agar. There two biotypes of *F. tularensis:* type A and type B. Type A causes more serious illness in humans than type B.

### 2. Transmission

The reservoirs of infection of *F. tularensis* are wild rabbits, squirrels, muskrats, beavers, birds, cats, dogs and sheep. This organism is transmitted to humans by bite of tick, deer fly or infected animal, by direct contact with infected animal, usually wild rabbit, by inhalation of aerosolized *F. tularensis* cells and by ingestion of contaminated meat or water. This organism is very easily transmitted to laboratory personnel and thus requires caution with its handling.

### 3. Pathogenesis

*F. tularensis* is a facultative intracellular parasite and is able to survive for a long time inside both phagocytic and nonphagocytic cells. Cell mediated immunity is primarily responsible for the control and elimination of tularemia. Anticapsular or anti-endotoxic antibodies play minor roles in the control of tularemia.

### 4. Disease Production

Tularemia features a number of forms: ulceroglandular, oculoglandular, oropharyngeal/gastrointestinal, pulmonary and typhoid. Ulceroglandular tularemia represents approximately 75% of this illness, and it is the result of a tick bite or direct contact with an infected rabbit. At the site of the bite, an ulcer develops with swelling of the local lymph nodes. Initial symptoms include sudden fever, chills, headache, generalized arthralgias and myalgias. Oculoglandular tulameria causes yellow nodules and very small ulcers on the conjunctiva following direct inoculation of *F. tularensis* into the eyes. Purulent conjunctivitis with lymphadenopathy of the local lymph nodes also occur. Oropharyngial/gastrointestinal tularemia results from ingestion of contaminated food, which leads to pharyngitis with lymphadenopathy or intestinal ulcers with mesenteric lymphadenopathy. Inhalation of *F. tularensis* can lead to pulmonary tularemia, which causes nonproductive cough, dyspnea, pleuritic chest pain, parenchymal infiltrates and cavitary lesions. Once organisms infect the lungs, they can enter the blood stream, which may lead to septic shock (typhoid tularemia). The mortality of untreated pulmonary or typhoid tularemia can reach 30%.

## 5. Diagnosis

A four-fold rise in IgG to *F. tularensis* between sera collected at the beginning of illness and 2–3 weeks later is believed to be sufficient for the diagnosis of tularemia. Indirect fluorescent antibody tests, enzyme-linked immunosorbent assays, tests for *F. tularensis* antigens in urine and intradermal skin tests are also considered useful.

## 6. Treatment and Prevention

The drug of choice for the treatment of tularemia is intramuscular administration of streptomycin or gentamicin.

Prevention requires protection from bites of ticks, deerflies via use of insecticides, wearing gloves when cleaning wild rabbits, proper cooking of food and vaccination. A live attenuated vaccine is recommended for laboratory workers, hunters, veterinarians or other individuals who are likely to be exposed to *F. tularensis*. Solid immunity follows tularemia. Committed lymphocytes, upon stimulation with specific antigens of *F. tularensis*, secrete a soluble substance which interacts with macrophages resulting in enhanced bactericidal activity for the tularemia bacilli.

## C. *Yersinia pestis*

### 1. Characterization

*Y. pestis* is one of the most virulent bacteria. The dose that infects 50% of experimental animals ($ID_{50}$) is believed to be 1–10 living organisms. It is a facultatively anaerobic, encapsulated, nonmotile Gram-negative bacillus with bipolar staining that gives the organisms a closed safety pin appearance.

### 2. Transmission

The natural reservoirs of *Y. pestis* are rats, chipmunks, prairie dogs, squirrels and rat fleas (*Xenopsylla cheopis*). Humans and other nonrodent mammals serve as occasional hosts. Plague is transmitted to individuals by bite of infected rat fleas, by contact with infected animal tissue or by inhalation of aerosolized organisms.

### 3. Pathogenesis

The precise mechanism by which *Y. pestis* causes illness is not known. However, there are five substances that have been linked with the pathogenesis of this organism: the F1 envelope antigen, which is antiphagocytic; the V antigen, which stimulates immunity in experimental animal and suppresses the synthesis of γ interferon and α tumor necrosis factor; endotoxin, which is apparently involved in the pathogenesis of septicemic plague and disseminated intravascular coagulation (DIC); a pesticin, which kills other bacteria; and an intracellular toxin, which is lethal for mice.

### 4. Disease Production

The incubation period of bubonic plague is 2–7 days. Onset is marked by fever and a painful bubo, usually in the groin or less often in the axilla. Without treatment, 50–75% of patients progress to bacteremia and die from septic shock within hours or days after the development of the bubo. Approximately 5% of patients develop pneumonic plague with mucoid and then bloody sputum. Primary pneumonic plague, that is, plague acquired by inhalation of aerosols containing *Y. pestis,* has an incubation of 1–3 days and begins with fever, malaise and a feeling of tightness in the chest. Cough, sputum production, dyspnea and cyanosis follow. Death on the second or third day of illness is common, and survival is rare without effective antibiotic therapy.

### 5. Diagnosis

Peripheral blood smears from septicemic patients or fluid removed from buboes stained with Giemsa or Wright's stain usually show characteristic bipolar staining of *Y. pestis* and provide presumptive diagnosis of plague. Definitive diagnosis requires isolation of *Y. pestis* from clinical specimens or demonstration of a four-fold rise in antibody titer against *Y. pestis.*

### 6. Treatment and Prevention

Streptomycin and tetracycline are the drugs of choice for both bubonic and pneumonic plague. However, meaningful reduction in mortality of plague requires prompt administration of these antibiotics.

Prevention requires short-term antibiotic prophylaxis for persons in close contact with persons with plague, use of protective clothing when at risk of exposure to rat fleas and use of insecticides and repellents. A vaccine composed of killed whole cells of *Y. pestis* is partially effective against bubonic plague but not pneumonic plague.

## D. Other Yerseniae

### 1. *Y. pseudotuberculosis*

Causes mesenteric lymphadenitis, which is a disease characterized by lesions ranging from local necrosis to granulomatous inflammation of lymph nodes, spleen and liver. The primary clinical manifestations are fever and abdominal pain that often resembles appendicitis.

## 2. *Y. enterocolitica*

The most common infection produced by *Y. enterocolitica* is enterocolitis, which usually occurs in children, and is characterized by fever, diarrhea and abdominal pain. It also causes acute mesenteric lymphadenitis similar to that produced by *Y. pseudotuberculosis*.

# XI. GRAM-NEGATIVE BACILLI WITHIN OR OUTSIDE THE GASTROINTESTINAL TRACT

## A. *Salmonella typhi* (*S. enterica* subspecies *enterica* serovar *typhi*)

### 1. Characterization

*S. typhi* is an encapsulated, motile, lactose-negative, Gram-negative rod. It is strictly a human pathogen.

### 2. Transmission

*S. typhi* is spread by the fecal–oral route most commonly via contaminated food or water. Human carriers are significant sources of *S. typhi*.

### 3. Pathogenesis

Opsonization and phagocytosis are inhibited by the *Vi capsular polysaccharide* of *S. typhi*. The ability of this organism to survive within macrophages by unknown means is another factor that contributes to the pathogenicity of *S. typhi*. Finally, the endotoxin of *S. typhi* may contribute in the production of fever, leukopenia, hemorrhage, hypotension, shock and disseminated intravascular coagulation (DIC).

### 4. Disease Production

*S. typhi* causes of typhoid fever, which has an incubation period of 3–60 days. The pathognomonic feature of typhoid fever is prolonged, constant high fever (40–41°C), which in untreated patients can last as long as 8 weeks, and it may be associated with severe anorexia, chills, constipation, weight loss, delirium, intravascular coagulation and the appearance of small, red macules ("rose spots"). Other possible findings include bradycardia (despite the high fever), hepatosplenomegaly or leukopenia and neutropenia. A number of possible complications, such as arthritis, bronchitis, hepatitis, meningitis, myocarditis, nephritis, orchitis, osteomyelitis, parotitis and pneumonia can also occur. Diseases that share some of the symptoms indicated above include rickettsioses, miliary tuberculosis, tularemia, brucellosis, leptospirosis, infectious mononucleosis and viral hepatitis. Three other serovars of *S. enterica*, that is, *S. enterica* serovar *paratyphi* A, *S. enterica* serovar *paratyphi* B and *S. enterica* serovar *cholerasuis*, cause a mild form of typhoid fever.

### 5. Diagnosis

Definitive diagnosis of typhoid fever requires the isolation of *S. typhi*, which is usually recovered from blood during the first week of illness. Bone marrow cultures often are positive despite the administration of antibiotics, and 75% of stool cultures are positive during the third week of illness. Measurement of antibodies to H and O antigens of *S. typhi* by agglutination tests (Widal test) are also useful. Titers greater than 1:160 to O antigen are usually encountered during acute typhoid fever. Also, agglutination tests for antibody to Vi antigen are more sensitive and specific than the Widal test.

## 6. Treatment and Prevention

Ciprofloxacin, ofloxacin, amoxicillin, trimethoprim-sulfamethoxazole or chloramphenicol is usually effective for the treatment of typhoid fever. The use of chloramphenicol, which has been the drug of choice, is not popular in the United States due to its association with the possible induction of aplastic anemia.

Prevention of typhoid fever requires good personal hygiene, suitable sewage disposal, chlorination of water supplies and prevention of known salmonella carriers from being food handlers.

## B. *S. enterica* serovars *enteridis, typhimurium, heidelberg* and *newport*

### 1. Characterization

They all resemble *S. enterica* serovar *typhi*, but they do not possess Vi antigen, and they are not exclusively human pathogens.

### 2. Transmission

Chickens, ducks, turtles and other animals transmit these serovars of *S. enterica*. Humans are infected by the consumption of contaminated eggs, unpasteurized milk or other contaminated animal products.

### 3. Pathogenesis

The mechanism by which these serovars of *S. enterica* produce disease is not known.

### 4. Disease Production

The most common disease produced by the serovars of *S. enterica*, which cause nontyphoidal salmonellosis, is gastroenteritis, characterized by fever and diarrhea. The disease is usually self-limited and does not need specific therapy. However, rare complications, especially in immunocompromised patients, can occur and may include endocarditis, cholecystitis, splenic abscesses, urinary tract infections, pneumonia and empyema, meningitis, septic arthritis and osteomyelitis.

### 5. Diagnosis

Isolation of salmonellae from stool, blood or tissue fluids.

### 6. Treatment and Prevention

For complications of nontyphoidal salmonelosis, ceftriaxone and chloramphenicol.

Prevention is difficult due to widespread distribution of the etiological agents. Thus, hygienic food preparation and quality testing are recommended.

### C. *Shigella dysenteriae, Shigella flexneri, Shigella boydii,* and *Shigella sonnei*

#### 1. Characterization

These organisms do not ferment lactose, are nonmotile, facultative anaerobic, Gram-negative rods that can be isolated on the selective *Salmonella–Shigella* agar plates. They can be differentiated from salmonellae in that they do not produce acid anaerobically from glucose or $H_2S$ from the metabolism of amino acids and they are nonmotile. Based on differences in their somatic O antigen, they are divided into antigenic groups A, B, C and D.

#### 2. Transmission

*S. dysenteriae, S. flexneri, S. boydii* and *S. sonnei* are human pathogens, and thus they are not found in soil or water without human contamination. They are transmitted from person to person by the fecal–oral route or by contaminated food, water, flies and fomites. Transmission may also occur by anal–oral sexual contact.

#### 3. Pathogenesis

Disease production by shigellae has been associated with the ability of these organisms to invade colonic epithelial cells, multiply in them and then spread from cell to cell without exposure to the host's defenses. The spread from cell to cell is accomplished by the polymerization of actin at the end of the dividing cell.

Another virulence factor for *S. dysenteriae* type 1 is the production of Shiga toxin, which by inactivation of the $60s$ ribosome inhibits protein synthesis and thus kills colonic epithelial cells. Finally, the endotoxin of shigellae contributes to the production of inflammation, fever, changes in cellular permeability, leakage of blood and tissue necrosis.

#### 4. Disease Production

Shigellosis has an incubation period of 1–4 days. This illness starts with fever, abdominal cramps, watery diarrhea that may progress to bloody diarrhea and dysentery. Dysentery features passing of stools with blood, pus and mucus 10–30 times a day. Patients with mild to moderate severity recover without specific therapy in 2–7 days. Severe shigellosis can lead to perforation of the colon, seizures or death. Symptoms of shigellosis resemble those produced by enterohemorrhagic, or enteroinvasive, *Escherichia coli, Campylobacter jejuni, Salmonella enteritis, Yersenia enterocolitica, Clostridium difficile* and *Entamoeba histolytica.*

#### 5. Diagnosis

*Shigella* is never a part of the normal human intestinal flora, thus stool culture is required for specific diagnosis. An enzyme-linked immunoassay can detect Shiga toxin in stools in 3 hours. Agglutination tests can also be used for the diagnosis because patients develop antibodies to O antigen. Cultivation of shigellae should be done on such selective media as the salmonella–shigella, MacConkey, Hektoen or xylose-lysine-deoxycholate.

### 6. Treatment and Prevention

Oral hydration solutions for mild to moderate cases of shigellosis; tetracycline and ciprofloxacin for severe cases with bloody diarrhea and dysentery.

Prevention requires care in the preparation and handling of food, proper personal hygiene and decontamination of water supplies and patient environment.

## D. *Escherichia coli*

### 1. Characterization

*E. coli* differs from the pathogenic species of salmonellae and shigellae in that it ferments both glucose and lactose. The somatic O antigens of the lipopolysaccharide (LPS), the capsular antigens K and its flagellar H antigens are used for serological subdivision and association with various diseases. For example, the 0157:H7 serogroup of *E. coli* is linked to the production of hemorrhagic colitis and hemolytic uremic syndrome (HUS). *E. coli* with K1 capsular antigens are associated with urinary tract infections, bacteremia and meningitis.

### 2. Transmission

*E. coli* is the most commonly encountered member of the Enterobacteriaceae in the normal colonic flora. It is usually transmitted by the fecal–oral route and generally involves consumption of contaminated food or water.

### 3. Pathogenesis

Many enteric bacteria are part of the normal colonic flora and do not cause disease. Illness requires the possession by the etiological agents of capsules, pili, endotoxins and exotoxins (enterotoxins). Immunosuppression will allow enteric bacteria that do not produce capsules, pili, endotoxins or exotoxins to cause disease. The function of capsules, pili and endotoxins has been explained previously. *E. coli* produces a heat-labile enterotoxin which activates adenylate cyclase, causing a rise in the intracellular concentration of cyclic adenosine monophosphate. This inhibits absorption of sodium and stimulates excretion of chloride. The end result is intestinal secretion, which causes diarrhea. The heat-stable enterotoxin of *E. coli* acts in a manner similar to heat-labile enterotoxin, with the exception that it activates guanylate cyclase rather than adenylate cyclase. *E. coli* 0157:H7 produces an exotoxin that resembles the Shiga toxin of the *Shigella* species. It is also known as verotoxin, and its mode of action is similar to Shiga toxin, that is, it destroys human colonic cells.

### 4. Disease Production

a. **Gastroenteritis.** The most common cause of gastroenteritis (traveler's diarrhea) is enterotoxigenic *E. coli* (ETEC) for adults and enteropathogenic *E. coli* (EPEC) for children. It has an incubation period of 1–2 days, it is due to the action of the heat-stable, or heat-labile enterotoxin, and it is associated with frequent and copious diarrhea and abdominal cramps which may last 2–4 days. The enteroinvasive strains of *E. coli* (EIEC) induce pronounced inflammation, fever and bloody diarrhea with leukocytes in the stools. This type of diarrhea resembles that produced by *S. dysenteriae* type 1. Other strains of *E. coli*, for example serotype 0157:H7, cause hemorrhagic colitis and are called enterohemorrhagic (EHEC). These strains have also been associated with the hemolytic–uremic syndrome (HUS) in children and in elderly individuals. The symptoms may include inflammation, hemorrhage, edema, necrosis of the colonic or glomerular capillary endothelial cells, microangiopathic hemolytic anemia, thrombocytopenia and renal failure.

b. **Infections of the Urinary Tract.** *E. coli* is the most common cause of infections of bladder, renal pelvis and kidney. This finding is partly explained by the large numbers of *E. coli* commonly found in the large intestine which contaminate the perineum and urethra, especially in women. Certain serotypes predominate in urinary tract infections. Properties associated with the virulence of these serotypes include possession of pili, which allow the organisms to adhere to uroepithelial cells, hemolysin production and the amount and type of the capsular antigen K.

c. **Meningitis.** Encapsulated K1 *E. coli* is the most common cause of neonatal meningitis, and it is a consequence of hospital-acquired septicemia. It should be pointed out, however, that with the exception of urinary tract infections, extra-intestinal infections caused by *E. coli* are uncommon when there in no breach in normal host defenses. Obviously, immunosuppression allows *E. coli* and other members of enterobacteriaceae to become potent opportunists.

## 5. Diagnosis

*E. coli* forms a unique green sheen on differential EMB medium and pink colonies on MacConkey medium. It can be differentiated from other lactose-fermenting enteric bacteria by its ability to form indol from tryptophane, give a positive methyl red test, use citrate as its sole source of carbon, produce acetyl methyl carbinol (positive Voges–Proskauer reaction), form flagella, and decarboxylate lysine. Finally the various serotypes of *E. coli* may be identified with specific antisera for the O, K and H antigens.

## 6. Treatment and Prevention

Specific treatment for mild diarrheal disease is usually not required. Bloody diarrheas and other extraintestinal infections may require rehydration, removal of necrotic tissue, pus, foreign bodies and use of suitable antibiotic treatment schedules. A wide range of antibiotics, such as trimethoprim-sulfamethoxazole, ceftriaxone, ciprofloxacin, ampicillin, aztreonam, imipenem or others are available, but due to incidence of plasmid mediated antibiotic resistance, antibiotic susceptibility tests must be conducted for effective antibiotic therapy.

There are no specific measures for the prevention of diseases caused by *E. coli*. Proper personal hygiene, avoidance of consumption of uncooked foods and contaminated liquids and chemoprophylaxis may reduce the incidence of enterobacterial disease.

## E. *Klebsiella, Enterobacter, Serratia, Proteus, Pseudomonas*

1. ***Klebsiella pneumoniae*** is an encapsulated, non-motile, indole-negative, lactose-fermenting Gram-negative rod.

   It is a normal inhabitant of the human intestinal tract, and thus disease is endogenous or acquired by contact spread. It is an opportunistic organism which may cause pneumonia (similar to that produced by *S. pneumoniae*) in immunocompromised, usually hospitalized, patients. Due to the incidence of multiple antibiotic resistance encoded by plasmids, effective therapy requires antibiotic susceptibility testing. Prevention rests on strict observance of hygienic hospital practices.

2. ***Enterobacter cloacae*** is a lactose-fermenting, motile, indol-negative, Gram-negative rod. It constitutes part of the normal intestinal flora and in healthy individuals is essentially nonpathogenic. However, in immunocompromised, usually hospitalized, patients it may cause wound infections or respiratory or urinary tract infections. What has been stated for *K. pneumoniae* concerning therapy and prevention is also applicable for *E. cloacae.*

3. ***Serratia marcescens*** is a late lactose-fermenting, pigmented Gram-negative rod which forms red colonies. It is found frequently in water from which it can be transmitted to humans; when they are healthy, it is essentially nonpathogenic. However, in immunocompromised, hospitalized patients it may cause sepsis, pneumonia and urinary tract infections with strains that are multi-resistant to many antibiotics due to carriage of plasmids that encode for resistance to many antibiotics. Disease production in immunocompromised, hospitalized patients is facilitated by such invasive procedures as respiratory intubation, manipulation of the urinary tract and intravenous catheterization.

4. ***Proteus mirabilis*** belongs to the family of proteae, a group of germs that includes the genera *Proteus, Morganella* and *Providencia*, which are opportunistic pathogens found in varying frequencies in the normal human intestinal tract, soil and water. *Proteus* and *Morganella* differ from enterobacteriaceae in that the species belonging to these genera produce a potent urease. *P. mirabilis* and *P. vulgaris* do not form confined, discrete colonies and tend to swarm over the surface of enriched culture media. *P. vulgaris* strains OX-19, OX-2 and OX-K share antigens with rickettsia of the typhus and the spotted fever group and are agglutinated by antibodies produced by patients with these rickettsial diseases (Weil–Felix test). *P. mirabilis* and *P. vulgaris* are essentially nonpathogenic but may produce hospital-acquired (nosocomial) diseases that involve the urinary tract, lungs and the circulatory system in immunosuppressed patients. What has been stated for *K. pneumoniae, E. cloacae* and *S. marcescens* concerning therapy and prevention is also applicable for *P. mirabilis* and *P. vulgaris.*

5. *Pseudomonas aeruginosa*

   a. Characterization. *P. aeruginosa* is an aerobic, oxidase-positive motile, Gram-negative rod with polar flagella, which produces the blue-green color (pyocyanin). It is not a member of the family enterobacteriaceae.

   b. Transmission. It is widely distributed in the environment, and it may be found in the gastrointestinal tract of some healthy individuals and in higher proportions in hospitalized immunocompromised patients. Thus transmission can occur exogenously, or endogenously.

c. **Pathogenesis.** *P. aeruginosa* produces an exotoxin A, which acts in a manner similar to diphtheria exotoxin, that is, it inhibits protein synthesis by ADP ribosylation of elongation factor 2. Extracellular slime production, especially alginase, by some strains in cystic fibrosis patients interferes with phagocytosis. Production of elastases and proteases facilitates the destruction of tissue at the site of infection. The endotoxin of *P. aeruginosa*—may also contribute to the pathogenicity of this organism. It should be noted, however, that *P. aeruginosa* is essentially an opportunistic microbe that usually causes illness in immunocompromised, hospitalized patients. Its ability to grow in water may result in the contamination of intravenous fluids, distilled water and inhalation and anesthesia equipment.

d. **Disease Production.** Most cystic fibrosis patients suffer from chronic pneumonia which eventually destroys their lungs. Cancer and intensive care patients are also good candidates for developing pneumonia. Intravenous drug users and diabetics, when immunocompromised, are prone to osteomyelitis. Debilitated individuals in hospitals and nursing homes have an enhanced risk of developing pyelonephritis or other urinary tract diseases. *P. aeruginosa* is well known for its ability to cause infections of skin and burns, which may lead to sepsis, endocarditis or death.

Given the right conditions, *P. aeruginosa* is an opportunistic germ that can infect any part of the human body, for example, corneal infections of contact lens users or osteochondritis of the feet. *P. cepacia* may also cause some of the infections indicated above in immunocompromised, hospitalized patients.

e. **Diagnosis.** The diagnosis of *P. aeruginosa* requires isolation of a Gram-negative rod with polar flagella which produces a green-blue pigment, is oxidase positive, lactose negative, utilizes carbohydrates only aerobically and produces colonies with a fruity, grape-like odor.

f. **Treatment and Prevention.** What has been stated for *E. coli*, *K. pneumoniae*, *E. cloacae* and *S. marcescens* concerning treatment and prevention is also applicable for *P. aeruginosa*.

## F. Vibriobacteriaceae: *Vibrio cholerae*, *Campylobacter jejuni*, *Helicobacter pylori*

### 1. *Vibrio cholerae*

a. **Characterization.** *V. cholerae* is a short, curved, comma-shaped, Gram-negative rod. It grows best at pH 7.0, but it can tolerate alkaline or salty environments. It is highly motile and moves by means of a single polar flagellum. It is classified on the basis of the O somatic antigen. Most of the epidemics are caused by *V. cholerae* O1, of which there are two biotypes (based on biochemical differences): the classic and the El Tor. Furthermore, *V. cholerae* O1 is subdivided into three serotypes (based on antigenic differences): Ogawa, Inaba and Hikojima.

b. **Transmission.** *V. cholerae* is a human pathogen, but the El Tor biotype survives better in salt water or brackish estuaries. Humans once infected can serve as vehicles of transmission. Usually infection is acquired from contaminated water, or sometimes, from food. Animals have not been shown to serve as reservoirs of infection.

c. **Pathogenesis.** The main virulence factor of *V. cholerae* is the enterotoxin (choleragen), which by itself can produce the symptoms of cholera. It is composed of the action subunit A and the binding subunit B. Once bound to human cells, enterotoxin stimulates adenylate cyclase, causing a rise in the intracellular cyclic adenosine monophosphate. This inhibits the absorption of sodium and stimulates the secretion of chloride. The end result is intestinal secretion, which causes diarrhea. Two other macromolecules have also been associated with the pathogenicity of *V. cholerae*. The first is a hemagglutinin-protease. This serves to detach the organisms from the small intestine, thus allowing them to spread to other parts parts of the intestine or assist in the excretion of vibrios in the stool. The second is the enterotoxin co-regulated pili (TCP), which facilitate the attachment of vibrios to bowel wall.

d. **Disease Production.** Cholera has an incubation period of hours to several days. It is characterized by an abrupt onset with vomiting and diarrhea. Voluminous fluid loss (15–20 liters/day) can lead to acidosis and hypervolemic shock with reduction of skin turgor, sunken eyes and cheeks. Remission or death can result in 2–3 days. Cholera is endemic in the Bengal area of India and Bangladesh. Death is due to dehydration and electrolyte imbalance. *V. parahemolyticus* produces a gastroenteritis with diarrhea following the consumption of fish or other seafood infected with this vibrio.

e. **Diagnosis.** Confirmation of cholera requires the demonstration of *V. cholerae*. That is, dark-field microscopy of the "rice-water" stools, biochemical tests and agglutination tests with polyvalent O1 antiserum. Isolation of this organism is made on the selective medium known as thiosulfate-citrate-bile salts-sucrose (TCBS) agar, where *V. cholerae* forms yellow colonies.

f. **Treatment and Prevention.** Immediate oral or intravenous replacement of water, base and electrolytes is of prime importance. Use of tetracycline or doxycycline is not required for cure but may reduce the duration of cholera.

   Prevention of cholera rests on chlorinated water supplies and appropriate sewage disposal. Whole cell killed vaccines are available, but they provide little protection.

2. *Campylobacter jejuni* and *Campylobacter fetus*

a. **Characterization.** *C. jejuni* and *C. fetus* are short, curved, comma-shaped Gram-negative rods. They are motile and move by means of a single polar flagellum. Campylobacters are microaerophilic.

b. **Transmission.** *C. jejuni* and *C. fetus* are normal inhabitants of the intestinal tract of cattle, swine, sheep, poultry, birds, cats, dogs and other animals, where they do not produce illness. Human disease is acquired from undercooked food or by direct contact with infected animals.

c. **Pathogenesis.** The mechanism of pathogenicity remains to be elucidated. Enterotoxins and cytotoxins may be produced by campylobacters, but their function is unclear. Motility and ability to attach to intestinal wall appear to favor disease production. Also the production of a proteinaceous surface, capsule-like, structure by *C. fetus* may protect this campylobacter from complement mediated killing and opsonization.

d. **Disease Production.** *C. jejuni* is a major cause of diarrhea in the United States. *C. jejuni*, enterotoxigenic *E. coli* and rotavirus are the three most common causes of diarrhea in the world. The enterocolitis caused by *C. jejuni* and *C. fetus* begins as a watery, foul-smelling diarrhea followed by bloody stools, fever and abdominal pain. The campylobacters may invade the blood stream and cause bacteremia, which most frequently occurs in immunocompromised individuals or in the very young and the elderly. *C. fetus* is usually associated with systemic infections. A very rare complication of *C. jejuni* gastroenteritis is acute neuromuscular paralysis, known as the Guillain-Barre syndrome. This is an autoimmune disease that is due to the production of antibodies against *C. jejuni* that cross-react the antigens found also on human neurons.

e. **Diagnosis.** Stool microscopic examination reveals many motile, darting organisms, blood and neutrophils. *C. jejuni* grows well at 42°C while other campylobacter species and stool bacteria grow poorly at 42°C.

f. **Treatment and Prevention.** Fluid and electrolyte replacement. Patients with high fever and bloody severe diarrhea of more than 1-week's duration should be treated with erythromycin. For systemic infections, antibiotic susceptibility tests should be performed.

Prevention requires proper cooking of food.

3. *Helicobacter pylori*

a. **Characterization.** *H. pylori* is a microaerophilic, urease-positive, curved Gram-negative rod with a tuft of polar flagella.

b. **Transmission.** Humans are the major reservoir of infection for *H. pylori*. Transmission occurs by the fecal–oral or oral–oral route.

c. **Pathogenesis.** The ability of *H. pylori* to attach to gastric mucosa and its strong production of urease have been closely associated with disease production. Urease produces large quantities of ammonia, which neutralizes the acidity of the stomach and allows *H. pylori* to multiply in an acidic environment that is usually lethal for many bacteria. Ammonia production is also inflammatory for gastric mucosa, and this inflammation can lead to ulceration of the intestinal wall or perforation of the stomach.

d. **Disease Production.** The fact that there is definitive association between infection with *H. pylori* and peptic ulcer disease, that peptic ulcers usually do not develop without infection and that elimination of *H. pylori* from the stomach or duodenum ushers in a significant reduction in the rate of ulcer relapse provides strong evidence that *H. pylori* is the etiological agent of most gastric and peptic ulcers. Epidemiological studies have also shown that gastritis precedes the development of gastric adenocarcinomas, and it appears that *H. pylori* may play a role in the pathogenesis of gastric adenocarcinoma.

The key symptoms of gastric and peptic ulcers are recurrent burning gastric pain that can be accompanied by bleeding into the gastrointestinal tract.

e. **Diagnosis.** Culture at 42°C of biopsy gastric mucosa specimens with subsequent isolation of urease-, catalase- and oxidase-positive organisms, which when stained with Giemsa or silver stains show curved rods. Detection of a rise in IgG levels against *H. pylori* in the serum of patients, which drops 6 months after treatment. Breath tests involving use of radiolabeled urea. If *H. pylori* urease is present, urea is hydrolyzed and radioactive carbon dioxide is detected in the breath sample. In this breath test, the patient drinks radiolabeled urea and then blows into a tube.

f. **Treatment and Prevention.** Treatment involves use of what is known as triple therapy, which includes administration of bismuth subsalicylate, tetracycline and metronidazole for 2 weeks.

## G. *Bacteroides fragilis, Prevotella melaninogenica, Fusobacterium nucleatum*

### 1. Characterization

These organisms are anaerobic, pleomorphic, with vacuoles and swelling, Gram-negative rods. *F. nucleatum* may also form long, slender filaments and fusiform rods. *B. fragilis* is unique in that its lipopolysaccharide does not contain detectable levels of lipid A.

### 2. Transmission

*B. fragilis, P. melaninogenicus* and *F. nucleatum* are part of the normal human flora of the intestinal, genitourinary, or the upper respiratory tract. Thus the source of infection is endogenous.

### 3. Pathogenesis

The organisms indicated above are essentially nonpathogenic at their normal habitat. Illness usually results when native host defenses and the anatomical barriers are altered by tissue ischemia, trauma, surgery, perforation of intestine or invasive diagnostic procedures, which can result in the spilling of microbes into the peritoneal cavity. Infections caused by Gram-negative anaerobic bacilli are seldom caused by a single organism; they are mixed infections. An anaerobic environment is essential, and in mixed infections aerobic organisms help the growth of *B. fragilis, P. melaninogenica* and *F. nucleatum*. Little is known about the virulence factors of these microbes. The capsules of *B. fragilis* and *P. melaninogenica* and various extracellular enzymes produced by *F. nucleatum, B. fragilis* and *P. melaninogenica* may contribute to the virulence of these organisms.

### 4. Disease Production

When the intestine ruptures by trauma, surgery, or other means, *B. fragilis* enters the peritoneal cavity and can cause abdominal, pelvic and liver abscesses. From these infected areas, this organism can spread to lungs, brain, bones, joints, skin and soft tissue and produce pneumonia, brain abscesses, osteomyelitis, arthritis, cellulitis or gas gangrene and necrotizing fasciitis. *P. melaginogenica* is usually associated with periodontal disease, and necrotizing pneumonias are induced by aspiration of sputum. *F. nucleatum* can cause abdominal sepsis, abdominal and pelvic abscesses, otitis media, aspiration pneumonia and periodontal disease.

### 5. Diagnosis

Gram stain, anaerobic culture. *P. melaginogenica* produces black colonies, and cultures of *B. flagilis*, *P. melaginogenica* and *F. nucleatum* have a foul odor. Fatty acid analysis of culture supernatants by gas–liquid chromatography. Specimens should be kept under strict anaerobic conditions and be cultured as soon as they are obtained from patients. They should never be refrigerated.

### 6. Treatment and Prevention

The drug of choice for *B. fragilis* and *P. melaginogenica* is metronidazole, but clindamycin, cefoxitin and chloramphenicol may also be used. Infections caused by *F. nucleatum* are usually treated with penicillin G. However, successful treatment often requires also surgical resection, drainage and removal of necrotic tissue.

Prevention of any endogenous infection is very difficult, but good surgical technique and suitable use of prophylactic antibiotics may prevent infections caused by *B. fragilis*, *P. melaginogenica* and *F. nucleatum*.

## XII. SPIROCHETES

### A. *Treponema*

#### 1. *T. pallidum* subspecies *pallidum*

a. **Characterization.** *T. pallidum* sbs. *pallidum* is a very thin (0.2 μm), spirochete with acute turns on spirals and tapered ends which give this organism a corkscrew-like morphology. Between the peptidoglycan layer and the outer cell wall membrane, this spirochete has six endoflagella known as axial filaments. Contraction of these filaments is associated with the motility of *T. pallidum* sbs. *pallidum*. This microbe cannot be cultured on artificial media. Oxygen, water, trace of heavy metals, detergents and sunlight rapidly kill *T. pallidum*. The organism may survive for 1–4 days when blood from infected persons is stored at 4°C in blood banks. *T. pallidum* sbs. *pallidum* is morphologically, immunologically and genetically similar to *T. pallidum* sbs. *pertenue* and *T. pallidum* sbs. *carateum*. It can be seen following silver staining, which increases its diameter, by dark-field microscopy or by immunofluorescence.

b. **Transmission.** More than 99% of syphilis cases are transmitted by sexual contact. Rare cases of syphilis are associated with blood transfusion or in utero transmission. Humans are the natural hosts for the etiological agent of syphilis.

c. **Pathogenesis.** The mechanisms of pathogenicity and immunity for *T. pallidum* sbs. *pallidum* remain unknown. What is clear is that this spirochete does not produce any toxins, enzymes, capsules, adhesins or other virulence factors that can be linked to its pathogenicity. There is no immunity after infection.

d. **Disease Production.** Syphilis is known for its large variety of clinical presentations and for its progression through the primary, the secondary, the early and late (tertiary) latent stages.

The incubation period is dependent on inoculum size, ranges from 3 to 90 days and averages 3 weeks. Primary syphilis features a papule at the site of inoculation which ulcerates. The local ulcer has smooth, heaped up margins and a crusted hard base, which is known as a hard or Hunterian chancre. *Haemophilus ducrei,* which is also transmitted venereally, forms a similar genital ulcer, but it has a soft base and it is called a soft chancre.

The syphilitic hard chancre, which is a single, painless genital, anal or oral ulcer, is usually accompanied by lymphadenopathy. Generally, the ulcer heals in 1–2 months, but the lymphadenopathy can remain for much longer.

From the infected lymph nodes, *T. pallidum* sbs. *pallidum* can enter the blood stream and produce systemic disease, which is secondary syphilis. It features papulosquamous rashes on palms and soles. On moist areas, the papules coalesce and form lesions, called condylomata lata. Secondary syphilis is also associated with hepatitis, aseptic meningitis, periostitis, fever and generalized lymphadenopathy. Secondary syphilis heals spontaneously, but it may recur in the first 4 years.

Latent syphilis is defined as the presence of a positive treponemal serologic test in the absence of clinical manifestations and a normal cerebrospinal fluid examination. This stage of syphilis is divided into the early latent, which begins approximately 1 year following primary syphilis, and late (or tertiary) syphilis 1 or more years after primary syphilis. In developed countries, latent syphilis is currently very rare; however, in poor countries latent syphilis is not a disease of the past. It has been estimated that about one-third of untreated syphilitic patients develop late syphilis. Late or tertiary illness is characterized by the development of neurosyphilis, which can be initially asymptomatic then lead to infection of sensory ganglia of the spinal cord (tabes dorsalis) and the cortex of the brain (general paresis). In tabes dorsalis the patient is ataxic, experiences paresthesias, strong pain and bladder disturbances. Patients with general paresis are hyperactive, have hallucinations, delusions, illusions and a decrease in their intellectual and communicative abilities. During late syphilis, patients may also develop cardiovascular syphilis, which is often associated with necrosis and destruction of elastic tissue, especially in the ascending and traverse segments of the aortic arch, resulting in aneurism or coronary aortitis. Finally, late syphilis may be associated with benign "gummatous" granulomatous lesions in the skin, mucocutaneous areas and bones.

In utero infection is called congenital syphilis. This illness develops when immunological competence of the fetus starts to form after the third month of pregnancy. This suggests that to a large degree the pathogenesis of syphilis is due to the immune response of the host.

e. **Diagnosis.** Direct demonstration of spirochetes by dark-field or immunofluorescence microscopy in the fluid obtained from lesions of primary and secondary syphilis, followed by serology. There are two types of tests for the demonstration of antibodies. The nontreponemal tests measure nonspecific IgG and IgM called reagins, which are directed against lipoidal antigen from either *T. pallidum* sbs. *pallidum,* or the interaction of host tissue with the spirochete. The most commonly used tests are the Venereal Diseases Research Laboratories (VDRL) and the Rapid Plasma Reagin (RPR) tests. The tests are inexpensive and, therefore, useful in screening large numbers of people. There are also important for following the course of the disease. The quantitative titer of reagins increases as the illness progresses and diminishes after treatment. Patients with autoimmune diseases, hepatitis B, leprosy, relapsing fever, infectious mononucleosis and malaria give false-positive reactions. Thus, positive nontreponemal tests must be confirmed by a specific treponemal test. The treponemal test of choice is the fluorescent antibody absorption test FTA-ABS. This is a standard indirect fluorescent antibody test. It uses killed *T. pallidum* as an antigen, the patient's serum, which has been absorbed with an extract of nonpathogenic spirochetes to remove cross-reacting antibodies, and fluorescein isothiocyanate-labeled antihuman globulin. The FTA-ABS test is positive earlier in primary syphilis and remains positive in more patients with latent syphilis than the VDRL, RPR or treponema immobilization test (TPI). The TPI test measures the ability of antibody in a patient's serum to immobilize live *T. pallidum,* This test is expensive and difficult to perform, but it is an important research tool and has remained a standard for treponemal tests. Another useful treponemal test is the microhemagglutination for antibodies to *T. pallidum* MHA-TP. This test employs *T. pallidum* antigens absorbed onto red blood cells that are agglutinated by serum containing antibody against *T. pallidum.*

f. **Treatment and Prevention.** Penicillin G for primary and secondary syphilis. For treatment of syphilis in patients allergic to penicillin, tetracycline, erythromycin or cephalosporin is recommended. A mild reaction known as Jarisch–Herxheimer reaction may follow the administration of antibiotics. It consists of fever, chills, myalgias, tachycardia and mild hypotension. This reaction subsides in a day.

There are no effective vaccines for the prevention of syphilis. Thus prevention requires use of condoms coupled with detection and treatment of infectious patients.

## 2. *T. pallidum* subspecies *pertenue*

*Treponema pallidum* sbs. *pertenue* is the cause of a nonvenereal disease called yaws. It features ulcerating papules on the exposed skin, is transmitted by direct contact with infected skin lesions, is seen in West Indies and Africa and the majority of patients are less than 15 years old.

## 3. *T. pallidum* subspecies *carateum*

*T. pallidum* sbs. *carateum* is the etiological agent of pinta. It features hyperpigmentation and keratosis of skin. Pinta is transmitted by direct contact, it involves exposed skin of all age groups and is seen in South America.

The characteristics, diagnosis and treatment of *T. pallidum* sbs. *pertenue* and *T. pallidum* sbs. *carateum* are similar to *T. pallidum* sbs. *pallidum*. The diagnostic tests for syphilis will also be positive for yaws and pinta.

## B. *Leptospira*

### 1. *Leptospira interrogans*

a. **Characterization.** *L. interrogans* is a thin, very tightly coiled spirochete with hooked ends that appear like button holes when the organism rotates. It can be stained with silver or Giemsa stain and is visualized with dark-field microscopy. It can be grown in a medium composed of peptone, water and serum.

b. **Transmission.** The natural hosts of *L. interrogans* are rodents, bats, dogs, cats, sheep, cattle and other animals. Leptospira are excreted in the urine of animals which serve as a reservoir of infection, especially rat urine. Animal urine containing *L. interrogans* contaminates food and water, ingestion of which can lead to human infection. The organism can penetrate intact skin and conjunctiva once attached to these tissues. Farmers, sewer and abbatoir workers usually acquire leptospirosis by direct contact with *L. interrogans*.

c. **Pathogenesis.** Following penetration though mucous membranes or the skin, leptospira enter the blood stream and localize primarily in the kidney, liver and central nervous system. The mechanism of pathogenesis is unclear.

d. **Disease Production.** Leptospirosis or Weil's disease starts abruptly with fever, gastroenteritis, myalgias and chills. The organisms in the liver, meninges, kidney and conjunctiva can cause jaundice, aseptic meningitis, nephritis and conjunctival suffusion, respectively. Renal damage is the most important lesion. Solid immunity usually follows an infection.

e. **Diagnosis.** Isolation of *L. interrogans* from urine or blood cultures. Demonstration of spirochetes with hooked ends by dark-field microscopy or staining of centrifuged urine sediments. Demonstration of four-fold rise of antibodies against *L. interrogans* in the acute and convalescent sera of patients.

f. **Treatment and Prevention.** Penicillin G or tetracycline for persons allergic to penicillin. However, to be effective antibiotics must be administered as soon as the symptoms of leptospirosis appear.

Prevention requires destruction of infected animals, protection of food and water from rat, mouse, dog, pig, cattle and sheep excreta and vaccination of domestic animals.

## C. *Borrelia*

### 1. *Borrelia burgdorferi*

a. **Characterization.** The borrelia spirochetes are larger and thicker than treponemes or leptospira, their spirals are also large. *B. burgdorferi* can be stained with silver or Giemsa stain and is visualized with dark-field microscopy. It can be cultured microaerobically in artificial media. However, with the exception of skin, cultures of clinical samples obtained from patients with Lyme disease are generally negative.

b. **Transmission.** Lyme disease is transmitted by bites of ticks infected with *B. burgdorferi.*

c. **Pathogenesis.** Lyme disease was discovered only recently, thus the mechanism of pathogenesis of this illness is unknown.

d. **Disease Production.** The organisms enter the blood stream and seed other tissues, especially skin, heart, joints and nerves. There are three stages of the disease with considerable overlap. However, not all untreated patients exhibit all three stages. Stage 1 has an incubation period of 3–4 days to 4 weeks and starts with the appearance of an intense circular rash that spreads out from the site of tick bite. The rash resembles a "bull's eye," and it is called erythema chronicum migrans, or erythema migrans, which is the hallmark of stage 1 of Lyme disease. However, about 25% of patients do not feature erythema migrans. Stage 2 sets in within days or weeks after the appearance of erythema migrans, and it involves the hematogenous spread of infection to many tissues, including the skin, where a secondary erythema migrans may be formed. Stage 2 is associated with lethargy, fatigue, headache, fever, chills, stiff neck, aches and pain for several weeks. Stage 2 is also associated with heart blocks, myocarditis, pericarditis, acute septic meningitis and cranial and peripheral neuropathies.

Approximately 50% of the untreated Lyme disease patients in the United States proceed to stage 3 of the disease, which is the late and persistent form of Lyme disease. Stage 3 features joint problems, especially in the large joints. Untreated patients who have the class II major histocompatibility complex allele HLA-DR4 tend to develop chronic arthritis with erosion of bone and cartilage in one or both knees.

e. **Diagnosis.** It is based on the recognition of the typical erythema chronicum migrans skin lesion, cultivation of *B. burgdorferi* from skin lesions, detection of antibody against of any 5 of the following ten 18, 23, 28, 30, 39, 41, 45, 58, 66 and 93 kDa *B. burgdorferi* antigens by western immunoblotting. Demonstration of *B. burgdorferi* DNA by PCR can replace isolation of this organism by cultivation.

f. **Treatment and Prevention.** Doxycycline, amoxicillin, cefuroxime axetil and erythromycin as alternative antibiotics. However, to be effective, antibiotics must be administered as soon as symptoms of Lyme disease appear.

Prevention rests on use of protective clothing and use of tick repellents when camping or working in wooded areas. Ticks must also be removed immediately from body surfaces.

2. *Borrelia recurrentis* and *Borrelia hermsii*

a. **Characterization.** Morphology and visualization are similar to *B. burgdorferi.*

b. **Transmission.** The natural hosts for *B. recurrentis* are humans, and transmission usually occurs by bites of infected lice. *B. hermsii* is transmitted by bites of infected ticks. On rare instances, transmission of both spirochetes may occur via blood transfusion.

c. **Pathogenesis.** The mechanism of pathogenesis of louse- and tick-borne relapsing fever (LBRF, TBRF) remains to be elucidated.

d. **Disease Production.** Both LBRF and TBRF are characterized by high fever of over 40°C which lasts 3–5 days and then by an afebrile period of similar duration. This cycle is repeated 2 times in LBRF and up to 10 times in TBRF. The fever curves are pathognomonic for relapsing fever. The relapses are due to antigenic variation of outer membrane proteins of the spirochetes. The disease is resolved when antibodies have been produced against all possible antigenic variants. These antibodies in association with complement lyse the spirochetes, and immunity is induced. The clinical symptoms besides high fever may include shaking chills, sweats, myalgias, arthralgias, dizziness, inability to sleep, scattered petechiae, tachycardia, nonproductive cough and other symptoms.

e. **Diagnosis.** Demonstration of spirochetes in Giemsa-stained smears of blood taken during fever. Also visualization of spirochetes in blood by dark-field microscopy. Agglutination of *Proteus* strain OXK by antibodies present in the sera of patients with LBRF and TBRF. Such tests are possible because *Proteus* OXK and *B. recurrentis* or *B. hermsii* have common antigens. Thus, *Proteus* OXK is used as an antigen because it is easier to grow than the spirochetes.

f. **Treatment and Prevention.** Erythromycin, tetracycline, chloramphenicol or penicillin. Mild Jarisch–Herxheimer reactions, similar to those observed during treatment of syphilis, can occur in relapsing fever.

   Prevention of LBRF depends on reduction or elimination of body lice by delousing agents, cleaning clothes and bathing and by avoiding crowding and improving socioeconomic conditions. Prevention of TBRF depends on avoiding contact with ticks, that is, use of protective clothing and use of tick repellents when camping or working in wooded areas.

## XIII. MYCOPLASMAS

### A. *Mycoplasma pneumoniae*

#### 1. Characterization

Mycoplasmas are very pleomorphic because they do not have cell walls and thus are resistant to penicillins or cephalosporins. They are the smallest bacteria and the only bacterial cells which contain cholesterol in their cytoplasmic membrane. They can be grown on artificial media containing cholesterol where they produce colonies which have a dark center with light periphery resembling a "fried egg."

#### 2. Transmission

*M. pneumoniae* is transmitted slowly from person to person by aerosols.

#### 3. Pathogenesis

The virulence of *M. pneumoniae* (Eaton's agent) is associated with the production of an outer surface protein known as P1, which allows this mycoplasma to adhere to mucous membranes of the respiratory tract.

### 4. Disease Production

*M. pneumoniae* is the main etiologic agent of a typical or "walking" pneumonia, which is often due to tracheobronchitis. The common symptomatology includes headache, coryza, chills and a sore throat. Severe pulmonary illness, such as pleural effusion, respiratory distress, lung abscesses and consolidation, is possible. Extrapulmonary complications may also develop. These include meningoencephalitis, aseptic meningitis, encephalitis, myopericarditis, congestive heart failure, erythematous maculopapular skin lesions and vesicular exanthems. Disease with *M. pneumoniae* may result in the formation of IgM autoantibodies, known as cold agglutinins, because they agglutinate human erythrocytes at 4°C. *Legionella pneumophila*, *Chlamydia pneumoniae*, *Streptococcus pneumoniae*, *Bordetella pertussis*, *Haemophilus influenzae*, *Franciscella tularensis*, *Coxiella burnetii* and respiratory viruses may produce symptoms which are very similar to those induced by *M. pneumoniae*.

### 5. Diagnosis

Detection of a four-fold rise of specific IgG and IgM antibodies against *M. pneumoniae* in acute and convalescent sera.

### 6. Treatment and Prevention

Mycoplasmas grow slowly, thus a 14- to 21-day course of treatment with erythromycin, tetracycline or doxycycline is recommended. There are no vaccines available for the prevention of mycoplasmal infections.

## B. *Mycoplasma hominis* and *Mycoplasma urealyticum*

*M. hominis* and *M. urealyticum* can be isolated from the genitourinary tract of normal asymptomatic individuals and cause opportunistic illness in adults and infants.

*M. hominis* has been associated with the production of pelvic inflammatory disease, salpingitis and infertility.

*M. urealyticum* may cause spontaneous abortion, premature birth and pneumonia in newborn babies.

## XIV. CHLAMYDIA

### A. *Chlamydia trachomatis*

#### 1. Characterization

Chlamydia are classified as bacteria because they contain both RNA and DNA, synthesize proteins, divide by binary fission and are susceptible to tetracyclines, erythromycin or sulfonamides. They are obligate intracellular parasites because chlamydia can not synthesize ATP. They have two morphological forms: extracellular, infective, metabolically inert elementary body (0.2–0.4 μm) and intracellular, metabolically active reticulate body (0.7–1.0 μm), which divides by binary fission.

#### 2. Transmission

*C. trachomatis* is a strict human pathogen, and persons with asymptomatic genitourinary tract infections serve as reservoirs of illness for *C. tra-*

*chomatis.* Transmission occurs sexually, by passage through an infected birth canal and, in case of trachoma by infected finger, fomite and fly-to-eye contact.

## 3. Pathogenesis

The mechanism of pathogenesis of *C. trachomatis* remains unclear. Uptake into host cells may be by parasite encoded surface proteins. The intracellular habitat and the changes from the elementary to reticulate body may assist the organism to evade host defenses.

## 4. Disease Production

There are 17 immunotypes of *C. trachomatis.* Immunotypes A, B, Ba and C produce trachoma, which is chronic conjunctivitis. Immunotypes D, E, F, G, H, I, J and K cause inclusion conjunctivitis, urethritis, epididymitis, cervicitis, proctitis, endometritis, salpingitis, perihepatitis and infant pneumonia. Immunotypes L1, L2 and L3 cause lymphogranuloma venereum.

a **Trachoma.** Results from repeated episodes of inflammation in the conjunctiva and cornea, which can progress to scarring and blindness. *C. trachomatis* causes more than 6 million cases of preventable blindness in Middle East, North Africa and India.

b. **Inclusion conjunctivitis.** Affects newborns who were infected during birth. The common symptoms include conjunctival inflammation, purulent yellow discharge and swelling of the eyelids.

Babies 1–3 months following delivery through an infected birth canal may also develop afebrile pneumonia, which features rapid breathing, cough and respiratory distress.

c. **Nongonococcal and Postgonococcal Urethritis (NGU, PGU).** Urethritis that is not caused by *N. gonorrheae* is called nongonococcal urethritis. *C. trachomatis* causes 20–40% of NGU and PGU. Patients with these infections may be asymptomatic or experience urethral itching, dysuria and a white, mucoid discharge. The main complications include epididymitis and Rieter's syndrome. This syndrome is thought to be due to an exaggerated cell mediated and humoral immune response to chlamydial antigens, and it involves skin, mucosae of genitals, eye and joints.

d. **Cervicitis and Pelvic Inflammatory Disease (PID).** The majority of women who harbor *C. trachomatis* in their cervix are asymptomatic. However, a thorough examination with a speculum will reveal mucopurulent cervicitis in 30–50% of cases. This infection may spread upward and involve the uterus, fallopian tubes, ovaries and peritoneum, causing PID. Complications of mucopurulent cervicitis (MPC) include scarring of the fallopian tubes, infertility, ectopic pregnancy, perihepatitis (Fitz-Hugh-Curtis syndrome) and endometritis. Lymphogranuloma venereum is another disease caused by *C. trachomatis.* The symptoms of this venereal disease associated with immunotypes L1, L2 and L3 include a self-limited local genital lesion that progresses to an exuberant and suppurative, granulomatous lymphadenitis that is followed by fibrosis and scarring. Systemic signs including fever, chills, anorexia, headache, myalgias and arthralgias occur during the suppurative phase of adenitis.

### 5. Diagnosis

Chlamydia form inclusion bodies in the cytoplasm of the host cells. Inclusion bodies are accumulations of elementary bodies. Thus, diagnosis of a chlamydial infection depends on the demonstration of inclusion bodies in stained cell scrappings obtained from the infected sites. Cell staining can be done with immunofluorescence or Giemsa stain. In exudates, chlamydia can be demonstrated with fluorescein-conjugated monoclonal antibody specific for chlamydial antigens. Detection of fluorescent elementary bodies confirms the diagnosis. Other diagnostic assays include isolation of chlamydia in cell cultures, detection of *C. trachomatis* nucleic acid by hybridization, ligase or polymerase chain reaction.

### 6. Treatment and Prevention

Uncomplicated chlamydial infections can be treated, but not eradicated, with a single dose of azithromycin. Doxycycline, tetracycline or erythromycin are also effective when administered for 7 days at their recommended dosages. The treatment of choice for neonates and infants is erythromycin. Sex partners should also be offered treatment with the antibiotics indicated above.

Prevention depends on early diagnosis and treatment and use of condoms for the prevention of sexual transmission.

## B. *Chlamydia pneumoniae* and *Chlamydia psittaci*

*C. pneumoniae* and *C. psittaci* cause pneumonia which resembles pneumonia produced by *Mycoplasma pneumoniae* or many other microbes. This list may include legionellosis, tuberculosis, typhoid fever, Q fever, common bacterial pneumonias, coccidioidomycosis, infectious mononucleosis or influenza.

*C. pneumoniae* spreads very slowly in closed populations from person to person by aerosols or very close human contact.

Acute and convalescent sera may be tested for *C. pneumoniae* complement-fixing antibodies.

The tetracyclines are effective against *C. pneumoniae*.

*C. psittaci* is a normal inhabitant of the respiratory tract of psittacine birds, such as parrots, canaries, parakeets and many other birds. Psittacosis is usually transmitted to humans by excretions of the respiratory tract.

The diagnosis of psittacosis can be made by isolation of *C. psittaci* and by demonstration of a rising titer of complement fixing antibody in the serum of patients with psittacosis.

The tetracyclines are effective against *C. psittaci*.

## XV. RICKETTSIAE

## A. Characteristics of *Rickettsia rickettsii*, *Rickettsia akari*, *Rickettsia prowazekii*, *Rickettsia typhi*, *Rickettsia tsutsugamushi*, *Coxiella burnetii*, *Ehrlichia chafeensis*

The rickettsiae indicated above are Gram-negative, nonmotile, small rods or coccobacilli. They are obligate intracellular parasites. They are classified as bacteria because they possess both DNA and RNA, ribosomes, their cell wall is similar to that of Gram-negative bacteria, they can produce ATP, they have macromolecular synthetic capabilities, divide by binary fission and are sensitive to bacterial antibiotics. However, in order to demonstrate many of the bacterial metabolic activities rickettsiae require host cell synthesized cofactors NAD and COA. Thus rickettsiae can only be cultured in embryonated eggs or in tissue culture. They stain poorly with the Gram stain but can be visualized easily when stained with Giemsa, Machiavello or Castaneda stain.

## B. Transmission

Table 3-1 lists the modes of transmission of the main rickettsial diseases.

## C. Pathogenesis

The mechanism of rickettsial pathogenesis has not been clearly defined. Most rickettsia produce widespread nodular, thrombotic and necrotic lesions in the small blood vessels and capillaries. Thus their key lesion is vasculitis, especially in the endothelium of the small blood vessels. Their virulence has been associated either with the production of phospholipase A, which lyses the membrane of the phagosome and thus prevents the fusion of the phagosome and lysosome, or with their replication in endothelial cells. The subsequent damage to these cells increase vascular permeability, which induces hemorrhage, edema, ischemia and hypovolemia, leading to reduced perfusion of various organs or organ failure. Endotoxin may also be involved in the alteration in cellular permeability, fever, hypotension, and intravascular coagulation. Recovery from an attack of a rickettsial disease usually confers a solid and lasting immunity.

## D. Disease Production

### 1. Rocky Mountain Spotted Fever (RMSF)

The most common rickettsial disease in the United States is RMSF. The early symptoms of fever, headache and myalgia without rash are difficult to differentiate from those induced by typhoid fever, leptospirosis, Gram-positive or Gram-negative bacterial sepsis, other rickettsial diseases,

► table 3-1

MODES OF TRANSMISSION OF RICKETTSIAL DISEASES

| Agent | Mode of transmission | Disease |
| --- | --- | --- |
| R. rickettsii | Tick bite | Rocky mountain spotted fever |
| R. akari | Bite of an infected mite | Rickettsial pox |
| R. prowazekii | Bite of an infected louse | Epidemic typhus |
| R. prowazekii | Reactivation | Brill's disease |
| R. typhi | Bite of an infected flea | Endemic typhus |
| R. tsutsugamushi | Bite of an infected mite | Scrub typhus |
| C. burnetii | Inhalation of infected dust | Q fever |
| E. chafeensis | Bite of an infected tick | Ehrlichiosis |

viral hepatitis, infectious mononucleosis, influenza or enterovirus infection. A rash appears between the third and fifth febrile days. The maculopapular rash usually appears first on extremities, moves centripetally and involves the entire body including the face, palms and soles. Early antibiotic treatment will prevent the subsequent development of cardiac dysrhythmia, respiratory distress, hepatic injury, stupor, delirium, ataxia, coma, seizures or death.

## 2. Epidemic Typhus, Brill's Disease, and Endemic Typhus

The epidemic typhus caused by *R. prowazekii* occurs suddenly, spreads rapidly and involves many individuals. Brill's disease is a recurrence of a mild form of typhus caused by *R. prowazekii* many years after the primary infection. It is thought to be due to deterioration of immune responses, which allows the dormant rickettsia in human tissues to be reactivated and begin to grow. Endemic typhus caused by *R. typhi* occurs continually in various regions. The onset of chills, fever of 38.8–40°C, headache, prostration and myalgias is sudden in epidemic typhus, Brill's disease and endemic typhus. In epidemic or endemic typhus, the rash appears first on the trunk around the fifth febrile day and spreads to extremities. This rash usually spares the face, palms and soles. Rashes are not encountered in Brill's disease due to the presence of antibodies against *R. prowazekii* from the initial infection. Early antibiotic treatment will prevent skin necrosis, gangrene, pulmonary involvement, renal insufficiency, stupor, delirium, ataxia, coma, seizures or death.

## 3. Scrub typhus

The illness appears after an incubation of 10–12 days. It begins with severe headache, high fever and myalgias. A dull, red maculopapular rash may appear on the trunk from the fifth to eighth day of illness. The rash usually forms an eschar at the site of the bite of mite. Early antibiotic therapy usually prevents the possible development of generalized lymphadenopathy, splenomegaly, central nervous system complications or heart failure.

## 4. Q Fever

The key sources of infection for humans are infected cattle, sheep and goats. These animals, when infected, contain high levels of *C. burnetii* in their placentas. At the time of labor, *C. burnetii* is dispersed as an aerosol and illness follows inhalation of rickettsia. *C. burnetii* is quite stable outside the host cells, but it is killed by pasteurization of milk, which can be responsible for subclinical human infections. Q fever usually features fever, extreme fatigue, severe headache, cough in 50% of patients with pneumonitis without rash, sweats, chills, vomiting and diarrhea. In general, recovery occurs even without antibiotic therapy.

## 5. Human Monocytic Ehrlichiosis (HME)

*E. chaffeensis* infects mainly mononuclear leukocytes, where it produces microcolonies known as morulae. Humans acquire ehrlichiosis by bites of ticks infected with *E. chaffeensis*. The clinical picture resembles that produced by RMSF. However, rash occurs in about 6% of cases, and mortality of untreated cases is approximately 5% instead of 20% for RMSF.

### E. Diagnosis

The diagnosis of the rickettsial diseases described above is made by indirect immunofluorescence assays. A fourfold rise to a titer greater than 1:64 or a single titer greater than 1:128 is usually necessary for diagnosis. Cross-absorption to suppress antibodies to shared antigens among rickettsia provides a specific diagnosis for a given species. Polymerase chain reaction (PCR) amplification of DNA from clinical specimens for a given etiological agent can also be used for the diagnosis of rickettsial diseases.

Strains of *Proteus vulgaris* OX-2, OX-19 and OX-K share common antigens with some rickettsia. Thus *P. vulgaris* OX-19 is agglutinated by sera obtained from patients with epidemic or endemic typhus, while sera from scrub typhus patients agglutinate *P. vulgaris* OX-X. This was discovered by Weil and Felix, and thus the agglutination assay is known as the Weil–Felix reaction. This reaction is not completely reliable, and it is not used in the United States. For example, sera of persons infected with *P. vulgaris*, *P. mirabilis* or *Pseudomonas aeruginosa* will agglutinate OX-K strains of *P. vulgaris* to titers greater than 1:128.

### F. Treatment and Prevention

The antibiotic of choice for the treatment of rickettsial diseases is doxycycline, which is usually given for 5–15 days. Chloramphenicol and ciprofloxacin can be used as alternative drugs.

Prevention rests on avoidance of tick, mite, louse and flea bites, by use of protective clothing and appropriate repellents. Protection against Q fever for laboratory workers, veterinarians, shepherds and abattoir workers can be obtained by vaccination with heat-killed *C. burnetii*.

# Medical Virology | 4

*Kenneth E. Ugen, PhD*

## I. INTRODUCTION

Viruses represent a unique and interesting infectious agent in the field of microbiology. In fact, there is some debate as to whether they even represent a living organism. This idea comes from the observation of their "parasitic" nature, i.e. viruses are completely dependent on other organisms for their existence.

## II. STRUCTURE AND CLASSIFICATION OF VIRUSES

In the 1880s, they had been grown in animals and plants as well as in bacteria. Later on they were described as being "filterable" agents, which were associated with diseases of plants and animals. The "filterable" nature of viruses, i.e. the characteristic that they could pass through filters which captured other organisms including bacteria, indicated that these "particles" were exquisitely small. Among the definitive properties of viruses are the facts that they (a) are the smallest "organisms," (b) have only one type of nucleic acid as their genetic machinery, i.e. only DNA or RNA, (c) are obligate intracellular parasites and (d) lack any synthetic machinery of their own, i.e. they rely on the host molecular and biochemical processes to supply the necessary "materials" for replication.

The major properties which are used to distinguish viruses from one another are (a) nucleic acid type, that is (i) whether they had DNA or RNA as their genetic material and (ii) the strandedness of the viral genome, i.e. whether it is single or double stranded, the type of polarity (negative or positive), whether the actual genome is linear or circular as well as the size of the genome in terms of kilobases; (b) capsid symmetry, i.e. helical, cubic icosahedral or complex; (c) the envelope, i.e. whether it is present or absent (i.e. naked); and (d) antigenicity, i.e. how well the component parts (proteins) elicit antibody responses or cellular responses. This is of clinical importance since it can determine whether potentially protective immune responses can be elicited against the viruses. Tables 4-1, 4-2 and 4-3 summarize the major structural and

► **table 4-1**

**DNA VIRUSES**

| Virus Family | Structure of Virion | Genome Structure |
|---|---|---|
| Adenovirus | Cubic, naked | ds, linear |
| Hepadnaviruses | Cubic, enveloped | ds, circular (incomplete) |
| Herpesviruses | Cubic, enveloped | ds, linear |
| Papovaviruses | Cubic, naked | ds, circular |
| Parvoviruses | Cubic, naked | ss, linear |
| Poxviruses | Complex, enveloped | ds, linear |

genomic characteristics of DNA and RNA viruses. In these tables, ss = single-stranded and ds = double-stranded.

The major component parts of viruses include (a) the envelope (present in only some viruses), which is composed of a lipid bilayer as well as proteins or glycoproteins; (b) matrix, which includes structural protein and enzymes; (c) capsid/nucleocapsid; and (d) core, which includes the nucleic acid component of the virus as well as other proteins.

► **table 4-2**

**RNA VIRUSES: NEGATIVE POLARITY**

| Virus Family | Structure of Virion | Genome Structure |
|---|---|---|
| Arenaviruses | Helical, enveloped | ss, +/− 2 segments |
| Bunyaviruses | Helical, enveloped | ss, +/− 3 segments |
| Filoviruses | Helical, enveloped | ss, − thread-like |
| Orthomyxoviruses | Helical, enveloped | ss, − 8 segments |
| Paramyxoviruses | Helical, enveloped | ss, − |
| Rhabdoviruses | Helical, enveloped | ss, − |

► **table 4-3**

**RNA VIRUSES: POSITIVE POLARITY**

| Virus Family | Structure of Virion | Genome Structure |
|---|---|---|
| Caliciviruses | Cubic, naked | ss, + |
| Coronaviruses | Helical, enveloped | ss, + |
| Picornaviruses | Cubic, naked | ss, + |
| Reoviruses | Cubic, naked | ds, 8–12 segments |
| Retroviruses | Cubic, enveloped | ss, + diploid |
| Togaviruses | Cubic, enveloped | ss, + |

Figure 4-1 shows the basic structures of enveloped and naked viruses.

In terms of nomenclature for viruses, this is determined by a panel called the ICVT, the International Committee for Viral Taxonomy. Two alternate systems have been devised for viral nomenclature. This first system provides the species, disease name and virus. An example of this system would be the designation human immunodeficiency virus. The second viral nomenclature system lists viruses by species affected, virus group name and number. An example of this nomenclature system would be human herpesvirus 6.

## III. VIRAL INFECTION

Viruses can infect cells and result in several possible infection scenarios. The first is productive/lytic infection. Much of the replicative nature of viruses was obtained from the study of bacteriophages, which are parasitic viruses of bacteria. Figure 4-2 shows the basic structure of the bacteriophage.

Figure 4-3 demonstrates the single-step growth of bacteriophage. The eclipse phase, which ends with the appearance of intracellular bacteriophage as well as the burst of replication, is shown.

In this situation the infectible host target cell becomes infected and produces thousands or more of virus progeny. The host then dies, releasing the virions. The newly released virions then infect many new cells, and the cycle is repeated, resulting in the continued perpetuation of the virus. The second infection scenario is latent infection: during this type of infection the host does not produce new virus and therefore survives infection. The viral genome either integrates in the host DNA or exists as an extrachromosomal replicative particle called an episome. Reactivation can then occur upon stimulation of the cell, which can include another infection or stress etc. Upon this reactivation the new virus is produced, after which the host cell usually dies. The final overall infection scenario is persistent infection in which the infected host cells can produce a low amount of virus while often surviving. Alternatively, the host cells may die but the virus that is released is often controlled by the immune system,

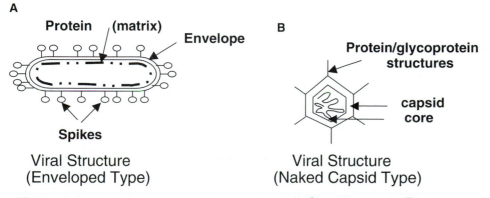

Figure 4-1.  Basic structure of the enveloped (**A**) and naked (**B**) viruses.

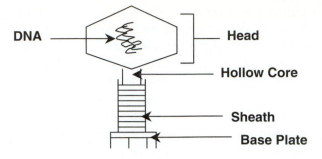

Figure 4-2.  Basic structure of bacteriophage.

which results in a low production of virus. The significance of persistent infections is that overall they are a major source of infections because the individuals infected are healthy carriers and can transmit infections readily and efficiently.

## IV. STEPS OF VIRAL REPLICATION

The overall steps of viral replication include (a) adsorption of virus to the surface of the host target cell, (b) entry and penetration of the virus, (c) uncoating, (d) production of initial (early) mRNA as well as non-structural proteins, (e) production of the viral genome, (f) production of late mRNA and structural proteins, (g) virion assembly and (h) virion release.

### A. Adsorption

In the adsorption step, specific proteins of the virion display specific attachment moieties that interact with specific host cell surface receptors which usually are glycoproteins or polysaccharides. Adsorption then occurs through the high-affinity interaction between the viral attachment proteins and the host cell receptors.

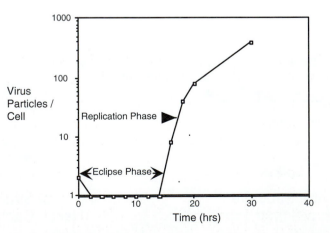

Figure 4-3.  Single-step growth curve of bacteriophage.

## B. Entry/Penetration

Entry is either receptor mediated for most naked viruses or through fusion of the virus envelope with the cell membrane for enveloped viruses.

## C. Uncoating

In the uncoating process the outer viral proteins undergo a partial degradation mediated through endosomal proteases. The virus nucleocapsid is then delivered to the site of replication. DNA viruses (except for poxviruses) will then be translocated to the nucleus, while RNA viruses (except retroviruses) remain in the cytoplasm. The viral nucleic acid is then available for transcription and translation for the generation of viral proteins.

## D. Production of Viral RNA

For DNA viruses the cellular RNA polymerase is used to produce the mRNA. In the case of positive-stranded RNA viruses, except for retroviruses, the genetic material is actually the RNA. Negative-stranded RNA viruses need to produce a positive complementary mRNA by the virion transcriptase. In the case of retroviruses, they require that their RNA be converted to DNA by virion reverse transcriptase. The DNA then integrates into the host DNA followed by the production of messenger RNA by the host RNA polymerase. The full-length virion RNA which serves as the genetic material of the virus is produced by the RNA polymerase of the host.

## E. Production and Role of Viral Protein

In a general sense, several types of proteins are produced by viruses: (a) immediate early proteins have regulatory functions such as modulating the host and boosting gene expression of early viral genes; (b) early proteins mediate viral nucleic acid replication such as DNA polymerase; (c) late proteins are utilized to form the viral particle of the virion.

Table 4-4 lists the major antiviral agents and their mode of action, which targets some of the types of proteins listed above.

# V. RESPIRATORY TRACT INFECTIONS OF VIRAL ETIOLOGY

Among the major medical conditions caused by viruses are the respiratory tract infections. The common respiratory tract viruses are as follows: (a) Orthomyxoviruses, which include the influenza viruses A, B and C; (b) Paramyxoviruses, which include parainfluenza virus, respiratory syncytial virus (RSV) and mumps; (c) Adenoviruses; (d) Coronaviruses; and (e) Picornaviruses, which include enteroviruses and rhinoviruses.

In general the infection of the respiratory tract is through inhalation or ingestion. In all there are greater than 220 viral serotypes that are associated with upper respiratory tract infections.

## ► table 4-4

**ANTIVIRALS: EXAMPLES AND MODES OF ACTION**

| Method of Action | Major Examples |
|---|---|
| Nucleic acid synthesis inhibitors | **Anti-Herpesvirus** |
| | *Nucleoside inhibitors* |
| |    Acyclovir |
| |    Ganciclovir |
| | *Non-nucleoside inhibitors* |
| |    Foscarnet |
| | **Anti-Retroviral (HIV)** |
| | *Nucleoside reverse transcriptase inhibitors* |
| |    Azidothymidine (AZT) |
| |    Dideoxyinosine (ddI) |
| |    Dideoxycytidine (ddC) |
| |    Stavudine (d4T) |
| |    Lamivudine (3T3) |
| | *Non-nucleoside reverse transcriptase inhibitors* |
| |    Nevirapine (Viramune) |
| | **Other Viruses** |
| | Ribavirin |
| Protease inhibitors* | **Anti-Retroviral (HIV)** |
| |    Indivavir |
| |    Saquinavir |
| |    Ritonavir |
| Viral protein synthesis inhibitors | Interferon |

*Prevents cleavage of precursor proteins.

## A. Influenza Viruses

These viruses, as indicted, belong to the group Orthomyxoviruses. There are three types of influenza viruses, designated A, B and C, which differ serologically and molecularly by their ribonucleoproteins. The A and B types are more severe, while the C type causes a form of the common cold. These viruses are single-stranded viruses of negative polarity and have an 8-segmented genome. Morphologically, they are spherical, enveloped particles about 100 nm in size with a helical nucleocapsid. The nucleus is the site of replication, and the major proteins are the hemagglutinins (designated H), neuraminidase (designated N) and the matrix.

### 1. Pathogenesis of Influenza Viruses

Overall, acute infections are characterized locally by desquamation of the ciliated columnar epithelium. Systemic effects are characterized by cytokine release. In terms of chronic infections and post-viral syndromes the role of immune responses and salicylates should be considered. Antibody responses to influenza viral proteins do occur. Antibodies to the hemagglutinin and neuraminidase protein contribute to neutralization of the influenza virus with those directed to the hemagglutinin considered to be the major neutralizing antibodies. In contrast, antibodies against the ribonucleoprotein are not protective.

### 2. Clinical Disease and Outcomes of Influenza Viruses

The incubation period for the viruses is about 2 days. The symptoms are characterized by an abrupt onset, fever, headache, myalgia and cough.

The infection peaks in 2–5 days, and the duration is usually 7–10 days. Complications can include pneumonia, and sequelae can also be associated with Reye's syndrome, cerebral edema, fatty degeneration of the liver as well as Guillain-Barre syndrome, which is characterized by peripheral neuropathy.

### 3. Epidemiology

Usually influenza occurs in the late fall through spring and is spread by inhalation of microdroplets as well as through the air and environmental surfaces. Epidemics of influenza spread from the east to west with an epidemic of A strains occurring every 2–3 years and B strains occurring every 4–5 years.

### 4. Antigenic Variation Among Influenza Viruses

Influenza viruses, like most RNA viruses, undergo considerable antigenic variation. This has considerable relevance for the occurrence of influenza pandemics as well as the development of vaccines against influenza viruses. The two major antigens of influenza of importance on this issue are hemagglutinin and neuraminidase. Influenza viruses usually change, through mutation and selection, their hemagglutinin and neurominidase proteins gradually over time, permitting them to persist in the population for a number of years. This gradual mutation in sequence is called antigenic drift. In addition, influenza viruses can also undergo major and spontaneous changes in their antigenic structure resulting from significant recombination between two different strains of viruses. These major recombinations, involving the hemagglutinin and neuraminidase proteins, are called antigenic shifts. These shifts are of relevance because they are responsible for the periodic influenza pandemics that plague mankind.

### 5. Laboratory Diagnosis

For diagnosis of an influenza infection the most suitable specimen is a nasopharyngeal swab. Serological diagnosis is most commonly done by ELISA.

### 6. Prevention and Therapy for Influenza

Trivalent inactivated vaccines are available the composition of which for a given year is based upon the previous years vaccine strain. In terms of therapy antivirals are only available against influenza A and these are amantadine hydrochloride (Symmetryl) and rimantidine which has a lower toxicity than amantidine. Non-salicylates such as acetaminophen are also useful as is other symptomatic relief in addition to bed rest.

## B. Paramyxoviruses

The paramyxoviruses include four parainfluenza viruses, the respiratory syncytia virus (RSV), mumps as well as measles. These viruses are distinguished by their glycoproteins, designated as HN and F. The nucleic acid is single-stranded RNA and with negative polarity and a non-segmented genome. They are spherical, enveloped particles about 150 nm in size and are characterized by a helical nucleocapsid.

### 1. Parainfluenza

Parainfluenza viruses have four major serotypes and are characterized by the HN and F glycoproteins. The incubation period for these viruses is about 1–3 days. These viruses commonly affect infants and young children and produce bronchiolitis and pneumonia. They account for approximately 15–20% of serious nonbacterial respiratory tract disease. Immunity to paramyxoviruses is transient, with repeated infections usually being milder than the primary infection.

## 2. Respiratory Syncytia Viruses (RSV)

RSV contains the HN glycoprotein but unlike parainfluenza viruses they do not contain the F glycoprotein. The incubation period is 1–4 days. Clinical symptoms include rhinitis, cough, fever, wheezing, respiratory distress as well as bronchiolitis and pneumonia, especially in infants. RSV can also cause croup. The illness can last up to 2 weeks, and the virus can be shed for up to 20 days. In terms of pathogenesis, the immune system appears to have a role the most significant contribution coming from IgE antigen–antibody complexes. The actual pathology of RSV infections involves the bronchi and alveoli in addition to there being necrosis of the epithelial cells. In terms of potentially protective immune responses (i.e. not involved in the pathogenesis), humoral IgG and secretory IgA are made. For laboratory diagnosis, a swab is the best specimen, which can be subjected to direct immunofluorescence, cell culture and serological analysis by ELISA. No commercially available vaccine is currently available, although several experimental vaccines are being evaluated. The problem of antibody enhancement of pathogenesis has created a difficult problem for vaccine development. In addition to an interest in vaccine development, treatment with intravenous immune globulin (IVIG) is currently under evaluation. In terms of anti-viral therapies, aerosolized ribavirin (Virazole) has been used with some success.

## 3. Mumps Virus

The mumps virus contains both the fusion factor and HN glycoprotein. The incubation period is 12–29 days with the average being 17 days. Parotitis, swelling of the parotid gland, is the most common manifestation. Mumps lasts about 7–10 days, with meningitis appearing in approximately 10% of the cases. Pathogenesis is not limited to the respiratory tract with the pancreas, reproductive tract as well as the CNS being affected. In the disease process, necrosis of the epithelial cells lining the salivary glands occurs along with concomitant inflammation marked by mononuclear cell infiltrates and edema. Antibody responses to mumps virus provide life-long immunity with some protective cross reactivity against parainfluenza virus. The infection is communicable 7 days prior to the onset of symptoms to 9 days after. Ages 5–15 are the most common age affected by this virus. For laboratory diagnosis specimens that can be used include nasopharyngeal swab, urine and blood. To establish diagnosis either direct immunofluorescence, cell culture (for detection of cytoplasmic inclusions) or serology can be used. An effective vaccine is available which has been used as part of the MMR (measles-mumps-rubella) vaccine since 1968. There is no specific antiviral therapy available.

The measles virus is covered under the section on Exanthems, Enanthems and Poxviruses.

## C. Adenoviruses

Adenoviruses are naked, icosahedral-shaped double-stranded DNA viruses in which replication occurs in the nucleus. There are 41 human serotypes with types 1, 2, 3, 5 and 7 being the most important. Clinically, adenoviruses cause pharyngitis and/or conjunctivitis, with pneumonia being a problem in the immunocompromised host. Pathologically, adenoviruses are spread by microdroplets and fomites and is characterized by necrosis of the respiratory epithelial cells and the occurrence of the intranuclear inclusions. Immune responses result in type specific antibodies with no cross protection against the other types. Epidemiologically, the infection is not seasonal. Laboratory diagnosis is typically made on a nasopharyngeal swab or eye swab if conjunctivitis is present. Detection can be made with direct immunofluorescence or cell culture using heterodiploid cell culture. A vaccine is available for the military only and is against types 3, 4 and 7.

## D. Other Respiratory Viruses

The rhinoviruses, which are naked single-stranded picornaviruses, are another significant cause of respiratory infections. It is one of the causes of the common cold. Symptoms of the common cold usually begin 2–3 days after exposure to the virus. There are over 100 different serotypes of rhinoviruses. Another group of viruses which result in a form of the common cold is the coronaviruses. These are positive single stranded enveloped RNA viruses which have petal like projections (corona).

## VI. HEPATITIS VIRUSES

Viral hepatitis may result from a spectrum of different viruses; however, there is a group of genetically unrelated viruses, referred to as the hepatitis viruses, which is responsible for the majority of cases of viral-induced liver inflammation. These may result in mild to severe acute disease as well as various forms of chronic infections.

The following viruses cause hepatitis with the abbreviation and group to which the virus belongs in parentheses: (a) hepatitis A virus (HAV, picornavirus); (b) hepatitis B virus (HBV, hepadnavirus); (c) non-A, non-B (NANB) hepatitis viruses, which include hepatitis C (HCV, flavivirus) and hepatitis E (HEV, calicivirus); (d) δ agent of hepatitis D virus (HDV, flavi-like virus); (e) non-A to E hepatitis; (f) herpesviruses including cytomegalovirus, Epstein-Barr virus, herpes simplex virus and varicella zoster virus; (g) rubella virus; (h) yellow fever virus; (i) dengue virus; and the (j) hemorrhagic fever viruses. All of the viruses that cause hepatitis fall within the range of 25–60 nm in size.

## A. Hepatitis A (HAV)

HAV is a positive single-stranded RNA virus with a naked capsid with cubic symmetry. It has been considered to be enterovirus-like and has only one serotype. In terms of clinical disease, hepatitis A has a relatively short incubation period of between 15 and 45 days. Most infections with HAV remain asymptomatic and can be established on the basis of specific IgG antibody. When symptomatic, the onset of symptoms is relatively rapid with anorexia, nausea and pain in the upper right quadrant. Frank jaundice usually occurs in less 50% of the cases but is more frequent in children and young adults. Some of the symptoms include dark urine and clay-colored stool with an enlarged and tender liver. Symptomatic cases are usually mild and last up to 2 weeks. Importantly, there is no chronic disease. The major pathogenesis of HAV involves replication in the enteric mucosa with associated viremia and spreading to the liver hematogenously. Many of the details of the pathogenesis of HAV are not completely understood. Immune responses to HAV result in the development of IgG which provides long lasting immunity. The epidemiology of infection includes transmission through the fecal–oral route as well as sexually. Cases of HAV infection are usually sporadic, but outbreaks from common sources do occur. Common sources for outbreaks include raw shellfish and contaminated water supplies. Laboratory diagnosis is through serology with acute disease being established with anti-HAV IgM; past disease can be shown through measurement of specific anti-HAV IgG antibodies. For prevention or therapy immune serum globulin can be administered to the household contacts of infected individuals. An inactivated vaccine available since March 1995 has been shown to be effective. Adherence to proper hygiene as well as other public health measures is important for controlling and preventing infections.

## B. Hepatitis B (HBV)

The infectious particle of HBV is approximately 42 nm in size, is enveloped and cubic and contains a partially double-stranded DNA genome. The hepadnaviruses, of which HBV is a member, are the only viruses which produce genomic DNA using messenger RNA as the template. This essentially is a reverse transcription process which is similar to that used by retroviruses such as HIV. The major proteins of HBV are the surface antigen (HBs), the core (HBc) and the e protein (Hbe). There are several serotypes, but they all share a common antigenic determinant. Importantly, the HBs protein is used for diagnostic purposes as well as for the successful vaccine development against HBV which utilizes a recombinant form of the surface antigen made through recombinant DNA technology. There is a long incubation period for HBV with which averages approximately 70 days. There is a more gradual onset of disease with overall more acute symptoms than occurs with HAV. Chronic disease occurs in about 15% of cases and results in a carrier state with persistent, active infection which can result in cirrhosis or primary hepatocellular carcinoma. The pathology of HBV infection involves necrosis of and immunopathological damage to the liver mediated by integration of the virus into the parenchymal cell nucleus. In terms of immune responses, anti-HBc antibodies develop relatively early, and overall the development of anti-HBs is associated with recovery; however, the persistence of HbsAg and HbeAg is indicative of a likely poor prognosis. The three methods of transmission of HBV are through the blood, sexually and from mother to child at parturition. The routine serological screening of HBV infection by blood banks has greatly reduced the rate of transmission through blood. Laboratory diagnosis of HBV infection includes detection of HbsAg as well as antibodies against Hbc. Additional testing can also include measurement of anti HBs, HBeAg and anti-Hbe. There is a "core window phase" during which HbsAg and anti-HBs are negative but anti-HBc are present. A successful vaccine against HBV, based, as indicated above, on recombinant DNA technology and targeting HbsAg, is approximately 95% effective; because of the association between HBV and primary hepatocellular carcinoma, the HBV vaccine can be thought of as the first effective vaccine against a human cancer. The vaccine consists of 3 doses, the first of which is given at birth. In addition, administration of hepatitis B immune globulin is recommended following exposure. Interferon has been given therapeutically for chronic hepatitis.

## C. Hepatitis D (HDV)

The hepatitis caused by HDV, also called δ hepatitis, is caused by a small single-stranded closed circular RNA-containing viroid. This virus is defective in the sense that it requires HBsAg for replication. The clinical manifestations of disease with infection by HDV is similar to that of HBV except that the likelihood of fulminant hepatitis resulting in death is greater with HDV. Epidemiological studies show that the groups high for risk of infection with HDV are those infected with HBV. Diagnosis of infection is made through measurement of the δ antigen or antibodies against this antigen. The vaccine against HBV can cross-protect against HDV. Likewise, HBIG can be used for prophylaxis against HDV for some liver transplant patients.

## D. Non-A/Non-B Hepatitis Viruses

Hepatitis C virus (HCV) is the major non-A/non-B hepatitis virus having clinical significance. It is flavivirus-like with an approximate size of 55 nm as visualized by EM. It is a single-stranded positive-polarity RNA virus. There are nine major genotypes and some subtypes. The epidemiology is similar to HBV and contaminated blood is the major method of transmission. Infection and clinical disease can manifest itself acutely and chronically. In the acute phase the severity of symptoms is intermediate when compared to HBV and HCV. Overall, 80–100% of individuals become chronically infected, and 25% or greater of those infected will develop chronic disease in 10 years or longer. Disease manifestations of HCV are the same as those of HBV including cirrhosis and primary hepatocellular carcinoma. In fact, currently cirrhosis due to chronic HCV infection is the most common reason for a liver transplant. Currently, the only effective and reproducible method for diagnosis of HCV infection is through serological analysis of specific anti-HCV antibodies. It is estimated that HCV has become the most prevalent blood borne pathogen in the U.S. Because of its established role in causing cirrhosis and hepatocellular carcinoma intense efforts are underway to develop effective vaccines as well as other therapies. Currently several experimental vaccines are being tested. In terms of therapy, interferon alpha has been used with some degree of success against HCV but only some of the genotypes appear to be susceptible to this drug.

## E. Hepatitis E Virus (HEV)

HEV is another non-A/non-B hepatitis virus. It is a single-stranded RNA calicivirus which is about 30 nm in size. The incubation period is between 25 and 60 days and transmission and disease is similar to HAV. HEV is clinically significant only in the developing Third World. It can result in 10–20% mortality among pregnant women.

## VII. VIRUSES OF DIARRHEA

Infection of the gastrointestinal (GI) tract by viruses is arguably likely the most common of all infections after upper respiratory tract infections. Infection of the GI tract may run the gamut from asymptomatic and inapparent (the majority of the infections) to fatal. In the developing world, between 5 and 10 million children die annually due to diarrheal diseases, making these GI infections of considerable concern from a public health perspective. Not all infections of the GI tract result in gastrointestinal disease, however. They may result in a systemic disease (i.e. hemorrhagic fever) or be limited to a distant part of the body (i.e. conjunctivitis due to enterovirus).

The viruses associated with GI disease are as follows: adenoviruses, astroviruses, caliciviruses, dengue, enterovirus, hepatitis viruses [A, B, non-A, non-B (C, E), δ D], Norwalk virus, reovirus, rotavirus, togavirus and yellow fever virus.

### A. Rotavirus

Rotaviruses are 11-segmented double-stranded RNA viruses approximately 70 nm in size with a double-shelled icosahedral shell. Four serotypes that have been recognized; replication occurs in the cytoplasm. Epidemiology indicates that infection is predominant in the winter months. Infection is most severe in children under the age of 2 years and is predominantly spread through the fecal–oral route. Rotavirus is a major contributor to infant mortality in the developing world, where it is responsible for nearly 1 million deaths per year, particularly in the malnourished and immunosuppressed. In developed countries such as the United States, rotavirus causes considerable morbidity but little mortality (less than 50 deaths per year) because of the widespread availability of supportive treatment to maintain fluid balance. With respect to pathogenesis and pathology, the virus localizes in the duodenum and proximal jejunum. This results in the destruction of the villus epithelial cells and blunting of the villi, resulting in mononuclear cell infiltrates and a transient malabsorptive state. The virus is shed for a period of 2–12 days, somewhat longer in the undernourished. The clinical course begins abruptly with vomiting for a period of 1–3 days followed by diarrhea for 5–8 days with a low-grade fever. Immune responses against rotaviruses are type-specific, with, in general, responses being long-lasting and with specific gut mucosal IgA being associated with protection. Rotavirus infection is very common among infants and babies, with 90% being seropositive for infection by 4 years of age. Breast fed infants have fewer problems with rotavirus infection because of IgA in the colostrum. Typical laboratory diagnosis of rotaviral infection involves detection of the viral antigen through latex agglutination and ELISA assays. Good hygiene is critical for the prevention of rotaviral infection, and electrolyte replacement for dehydration resulting from the diarrhea is critical to decrease morbidity and mortality. An efficacious vaccine was put on the market in 1999 but was removed shortly thereafter because of incidences of intestinal intussusception being linked to the use of the vaccine.

## B. Norwalk Virus

Norwalk viruses are small (approximately 35 nm), round, naked single-stranded RNA viruses that share similarity with caliciviruses. The epidemiology of Norwalk virus infection involves transmission predominantly through the fecal–oral route and involves contaminated water supplies and foods, especially shellfish. Family and community outbreaks are common, and, unlike rotavirus, infections with rotavirus are not limited predominantly to babies and children. The incubation period for Norwalk virus infection is 10–48 hours, followed by abrupt onset of symptoms, most notably vomiting and diarrhea. In general, the clinical symptoms of Norwalk virus infection is usually milder than rotavirus. The typical duration of symptoms is 1–2 days, and some respiratory symptoms are possible. The pathogenesis and pathology of Norwalk virus is similar to that of rotavirus except shorter in duration, with virus being shed for 3–4 days in the feces. Antibody is produced against Norwalk virus, but it is not protective with the possibility of disease recurrence. Studies indicate that approximately 50% of individuals are seropositive for Norwalk virus by middle age.

Diagnosis of infection is by ELISA or electron microscopy. The only preventative measures are good hygienic practices. There is no specific therapy or vaccine available.

## C. Enteric Adenoviruses

There are a number of types of adenoviruses that cause diarrhea, including types 38, 40 and 41. These viruses account for approximately 5–15% of viral diarrheas in young children.

## VIII. HERPESVIRUSES

Table 4-5 lists the various types of human herpesviruses. Herpesviruses are large, enveloped cubical viruses with a double-stranded linear DNA genome. The lytic replication of herpesviruses is characterized by sequential expression of the immediate early, early and late classes of genes. The acute phase of infection in patients is often associated with herpetic

### ▶ table 4-5

**HUMAN HERPESVIRUSES**

| Designation | Common Name | Abbreviation | Subfamily |
|---|---|---|---|
| HHV 1 | Herpes simplex virus 1 | HSV1 | α |
| HHV 2 | Herpes simplex Virus 2 | HSV2 | α |
| HHV 3 | Varicella zoster | VZV | α |
| HHV 4 | Epstein Barr virus | EBV | γ |
| HHV 5 | Cytomegalovirus | CMV | β |
| HHV 6 | Human Herpesvirus 6 | HHV6 | β |
| HHV 7 | Human Herpesvirus 7 | HHV7 | β |
| HHV 8 | Kaposi's sarcoma herpesvirus | KSHV | γ |

(i.e. vesicular) lesions of the skin and mucous membranes. After this acute phase of infection, herpesviruses usually establish life-long latency in neurons or lymphocytes. The latent herpesviruses can become reactivated, causing herpetic lesions. Primary infection or reactivation of latent virus in immunocompromised patients is a life-threatening condition. The antiviral drugs acyclovir and ganciclovir can selectively inhibit the synthesis of viral DNA of some herpesviruses. Herpesviruses are large enveloped cubical viruses with a large double-stranded DNA genome. Infection is characterized by a primary phase followed by latency. When reactivation occurs, it is typically less severe than the primary infection, unless it occurs in immunocompromised patient.

## A. Herpes Simplex Viruses (HSV)

HSVs are characterized by sequential production of proteins (a) the immediate early proteins which transactivate early genes and down-regulate cellular genes, (b) early proteins such as DNA polymerase and thymidine kinase, which are required for DNA synthesis, and (c) late proteins that are assembled into new virions.

HSV-1 and HSV-2 undergo rapid replication in many different cell types; latency occurs in the nucleus of sensory neurons. In most cases HSV-1 infection is asymptomatic. Acute primary infection can occur in region of the head, resulting in pharyngitis, gingivostomatitis, herpes labialis as well as keratitis. The spread of this acute infection can result in encephalitis as well as eczema herpeticum. Reactivation of the viral infection can result in recurrent cold sores. An immunocompromised state of the patient increases the likelihood of severe disseminated disease. With HSV-2 infection, genital herpes can occur either asymptomatically or symptomatically as well as the neonatal genital herpes syndrome, which can be fatal. Overall, HSV-2 and HSV-1 are responsible for 90% and 10% of all genital herpes infections, respectively. Transmission of the HSVs occurs through direct contact with asymptomatic carriers. Latency develops after primary infection of the skin, which subsequently results in virus traveling through the axons to the nuclei of the ganglion. Reactivation of virus infection is, in effect, essentially a reversal of the latency process. Both thymidine kinase as well as the latency associated transcript (LAT) are required for the activation process.

Pathological manifestations of infection involves necrosis and inflammation resulting in macules, papules, vesicles, pustules and ulcers. Lesions can be noted on the skin and mucous membranes. Neurological manifestations can be characterized by necrotizing lesions in the temporal lobes. Immune responses occur against herpesvirus infections at least partially. Re-infection with a new strain is possible. Cellular immune responses are thought to be critical for the development of protection.

Epidemiologically, herpesvirus infections occur worldwide, with HSV-2 being primarily sexually transmitted. Diagnosis of herpesvirus infection is by physical examination, the Tzanck reaction as well as virus isolation. Treatment for herpes infections entails acyclovir as well as derivatives of this drug, including famciclovir and valacyclovir.

## B. Varicella Zoster Virus (VZV)

VZV is genetically similar to herpes viruses and results in latency in neurons. The diseases produced by varicella zoster include chickenpox, herpes zoster, disseminated zoster in immunocompromised individuals as well as post-herpetic neuralgia. The pathogenesis of varicella zoster infection begins with transmission by the respiratory route. This is followed by infection of the mucosa, local replication, a viremia, spleen/liver involvement followed by spread to the skin. This is then followed by a febrile state with a rash on the back of the head, ears, face, next trunk and extremities. As with many viral infections, severe disseminated disease can occur in the immunosuppressed. Reactivation can occur in the dermatomes, which results in a condition known as shingles. Epidemiologically, infection with VZV occurs worldwide, with over 90% of the population being infected by age 10 with this highly contagious virus. The development of cellular immune responses is responsible for clearance and the development of life-long immunity.

Diagnosis of infection is based upon the development of clinical symptoms as well as the presence of syncytia and intranuclear inclusions in smears. A live attenuated vaccine is available, but it is not safe for use in immunosuppressed children. In immunocompromised children a preventative high-titer IgG can be administered within 72 hours of exposure along with administration of acyclovir or analogues. In general, treatment is not indicated for uncomplicated cases of varicella, although treatment of immunocompromised children with the appropriate antivirals is indicated.

## C. Epstein-Barr Virus (EBV)

EBV is a B cell specific oncogenic virus characterized by latency and limited replication in the epithelial cells of the oropharynx. The Epstein-Barr nuclear antigens (EBNA) and latent membrane proteins (LMP) are unique to EBV and are involved in oncogenesis. The pathogenesis of EBV is as follows: (a) primary infection occurs in the oropharynx followed by (b) spread to and immortalization and proliferation of B cells; (c) activation of T cells; (d) immunosuppression with swollen lymph nodes, spleen and liver. Disease manifestations of EBV are (a) infectious mononucleosis, which is characterized by high fever, malaise, pharyngitis, lymphadenopathy, splenomegaly and hepatitis. Infectious mononucleosis is also characterized by the presence of Downey cells, which are activated T cells, which appear as atypical lymphocytes in the peripheral blood (i.e. mononucleosis); (b) Burkitt's lymphoma which is a B cell tumor of children in Africa. It is characterized by a *myc* gene translocation; (c) post-transplant, AIDS associated B cell lymphomas, which are oligo-/polyclonal B cell tumors with no *myc* gene translocation; (d) Hodgkin's lymphoma—evidence suggests a role for EBV in this malignancy due to the large number of EBV-positive cells present; (e) nasopharyngeal carcinoma—this malignancy has a relatively high incidence in China, and environmental factors are thought to be important. Epidemiologically, EBV infection is spread by saliva (often through kissing) and other contaminated objects. Studies indicate that approximately 70% of individuals under the age of 30 in the U.S. have been infected by EBV. Virus shedding occurs in asymptomatic carriers. Diagnosis of EBV infection can be made at several levels using different methods. These include (a) lymphocytosis characterized by atypical lymphocytes; (b) nonspecific antibodies which agglutinate sheep erythrocytes; (c) IgM antibodies to capsid proteins and (d) rising antibody levels against EBNA which is the most specific. Life-long immunity is developed against EBV after infection. No treatment is available because latent viral DNA is unaffected by any antiviral agents. An experimental subunit vaccine is being currently being studied.

### D. Cytomegalovirus (CMV)

CMV is a β herpesvirus and is characterized by latency in monocytic bone marrow cells; it also can infect lymphocytes as well as other cells. After primary infection CMV spreads to lymphocytes, spleen, liver, heart and the CNS. Subacute infection is followed by latency. Infection is associated with strong immunosuppression. The diseases associated with CMV infection are (a) congenital infection which occurs before birth through the placenta. This infection can be very severe, especially if the mother has a primary infection; (b) infectious mononucleosis, which can occur from sexual contact, and (c) a generalized type of infection which is associated with immunosuppression; this can occur with organ transplantation or AIDS and can result in CNS involvement, pneumonia, retinitis, colitis as well as organ rejection.

Cellular immunity is essential for controlling CMV infection. Approximately 50% of the U.S. population is seropositive for CMV infection. Methods of transmission include congenital, oral, sexual, blood transfusion and organ transplantation. Histologically, diagnosis can be made by the observation of enlarged infected cells and basophilic nuclear inclusion bodies. Other methods of diagnosis include immunohistochemistry, PCR as well as the development of IgM antibodies. Antiviral treatment regimens for CMV involve ganciclovir and cidofovir. Prevention of infection involves the screening of blood and organ donors.

### E. HHV6 and HHV7

These herpesviruses belong to the β group and are related to CMV. Infection by these viruses occurs in the very young, and T cells appear to be the site of latency. Cell mediated immunity is the major type of immune response elicited against these viruses. HHV6 is a ubiquitous virus that is the cause of a childhood rash known as exanthema subitum (also known as fifth disease or roseola infantum). There has also been some suggestion that HHV6 may have a role in multiple sclerosis, lymphomas as well as potentially being a co-factor for AIDS. HHV8 is also called the Kaposi's sarcoma associated herpesvirus. This is a γ herpesvirus, which is lymphotropic in nature and is related to simian oncogenic virus as well as EBV. Transmission is through sexual contact. Primary infection is not known for this virus, and latency occurs in B cells. Reactivation occurs with the production of tumors, particularly in the skin. These skin tumors are known as Kaposi's sarcoma and have been relatively benign tumors in males 65 years of age and older. These tumors have assumed greater clinical significance with the AIDS pandemic and are a frequent malignancy among AIDS patients. Anti-retroviral therapy in AIDS patients results in regression of the tumors. Ganciclovir has been shown to prevent tumor development but has no effect on existing tumors.

# IX. ENTEROVIRUSES

Enteroviruses are part of the picornaviridae family and comprise at least 72 serotypes including coxsackieviruses groups A (23 serotypes) and B (6 serotypes); ECHO viruses (31 serotypes); polioviruses (3 serotypes) and enteroviruses (5 serotypes). The enterovirus particles are single-stranded RNA with positive polarity. They are naked, icosahedral virions with diameters of 22–30 nm. Replication occurs in the cytoplasm. The host range is limited to primates except for coxsackieviruses. On an epidemiological basis the incubation period is between 2 and 10 days. The most frequent period for infection is from summer to fall, but this may be extended in tropical and subtropical areas. The virus typically persists in the oropharynx for 1–4 weeks and in the feces for up to 18 weeks, and transmission is usually through the fecal–oral route.

With respect to pathogenesis the infection of the gastrointestinal (GI) tract is followed by a first wave of viremia. The second wave of viremia affects the CNS and other organs. The lytic effects of the virus cause tissue damage and necrosis. In addition, inflammatory perivascular infiltrates become apparent. Clinical disease associated with enterovirus infection runs the complete gamut from subclinical to mild disease to pathology, which is life threatening. The lytic enteroviral diseases can be manifested as poliomyelitis, aseptic meningitis, encephalitis as well as acute respiratory disease. They can also be associated with immunopathologic and autoimmune disease such as myopericarditis, nephritis and myositis. The generation of neutralizing antibodies is important for recovery from as well as protection. Furthermore, IgA in the gut is important for protection. For laboratory diagnosis of enteroviruses, a throat swab or a stool or rectal swab is required. The virus can then be cultured in monkey kidney cells or human fibroblasts. Serology is usually performed only after the isolation of the virus. For the enteroviruses, vaccines exist only for poliomyelitis. In general, prevention of enterovirus infections is through good personal hygiene, and proper waste disposal is important. There is no direct therapy for these infections, and only symptomatic relief and supportive therapy is available.

## A. Polioviruses

There are three serotypes that exist for poliovirus, with the risk of paralytic polio increasing with age. Overall, approximately 1% of natural polio infections lead to paralytic polio. The virus gets into the CNS through the blood–brain barrier. In terms of clinical disease and outcomes, 90% of poliovirus infections are subclinical. The incubation period is usually 1–2 weeks. The types of diseases associated with poliovirus infections are abortive poliomyelitis, aseptic meningitis and paralytic poliomyelitis with asymmetric flaccid paralysis as well as bulbar polio. Prevention of disease produced by polioviruses through vaccines has been one of the great success stories in medicine. The Salk vaccine, which was first used in 1955, consisted of a 4-dose inactivated vaccine, which subsequently has been designated IPV (inactivated polio vaccine). The Sabin vaccine, which has been available since 1962, is a live attenuated vaccine preparation which has been designated OPV (oral polio vaccine). The drawback of using OPV is that there is a risk of vaccine associated polio which has occurred. Currently, the endemic sites of polio in North America is near zero, and there is a declining incidence worldwide. It is likely that within the next several years polio will be eradicated. The eradication of the virus will ultimately occur because of the generation of better inactivated, subunit and attenuated vaccines, the eradication of polio as a disease as well as the elimination of the vector for the poliovirus.

## B. Coxsackieviruses

Unlike polio, disease associated with coxsackieviruses is limited to the meninges and is characterized by exanthems that mimic rubella. The major diseases associated with coxsackievirus infection are coxsackie B myocarditis and epidemic myalgia.

## X. EXANTHEMS, ENANTHEMS AND POXVIRUSES

Exanthems (external rashes) and enanthems (internal rashes) are caused by a variety of viruses within several viral groups. These may, in general, present in several forms including macular, popular, vesicular and pustular or as a combination, i.e. maculopapular. Some rashes progress from one stage to another, i.e. from macular to popular. Frequently, a rash may be characteristic of a particular virus both in the form of the rash and its distribution over the body surfaces. However, many types of rashes present in a similar manner, and the causative agent cannot be determined based upon the clinical presentation. The viruses associated with exanthems are as follows: rubeola (measles), rubella (German measles), parvovirus B19 (fifth disease), human herpesvirus 6 (HHV6: roseola), enteroviruses (rubella-like rash), herpes simplex virus, varicella zoster virus, variola (smallpox) and molluscum contagiosum (pox).

## A. Rubeola

Rubeola is the 5-day measles. It is a paramyxovirus which falls specifically under the morbilliviruses. The incubation period is 7–18 days with a mean being 10 days. Clinically the disease is characterized by cough, coryza, conjunctivitis, fever as well as lymphadenopathy. Koplik's spots are enanthems which are gray-white spots surrounded by erythema on the buccal mucosa of the molars. These spots are pathognomonic for rubeola. The maculopapular rash is distributed centripetally and is semi-confluent and lasts about 3–5 days. Clinical disease is especially severe in immunocompromised individuals. In the developing world, the fatality rate is 15–25%. There is also bacterial superinfection in about 5–15% of the cases. This infection causes transient immune suppression. The pathogenesis of infection includes infection and replication in the upper respiratory tract mucosal epithelium, followed by viremia to the lymphatic and the B and T lymphocytes. The onset of the rash is associated with antibody production; virus specific cell mediated immunity also develops. Overall immune responses result in the development of life-long immunity. Epidemiologically, the peak occurrence is in winter and spring. Rubeola is highly infectious; 85–95% of those who are exposed get infected. Currently the most common occurrence of rubeola is in adolescents who have failed proper vaccination, but the disease can be devastating in virgin populations where there has not been exposure to the virus. Diagnosis is by clinical picture, i.e. Koplik's spots, or by serology (ELISA), direct immunofluorescence and cell culture. For prevention, a live attenuated vaccine, which has been available since 1965, has been very effective. The vaccine is typically administered at 15 months and 4–6 years or at 5 months and 15 months in endemic areas.

## B. Rubella

Rubella is a single-stranded positive-polarity enveloped RNA virus that belongs to the togaviruses. The infection which it causes is called the German measles (3-day measles). Clinical disease is characterized by an incubation period of 14–21 days. Manifestations include mild upper respiratory tract infection (URTI) and lymphadenopathy, with a macular rash on the head, neck and trunk occurring 1–3 days after the onset of the URTI. Congenital rubella infection can also be problematic because it is teratogenic when acquired during the first trimester. Winter and spring are the most common times for infection to occur. Diagnosis of infection can be made by cell culture or serology by ELISA. Prevention is dependent upon vaccination with a live attenuated virus, which is administered together with vaccines against mumps and measles.

## C. Parvovirus B19

Parvovirus B19 is a positive- or negative-polarity single-stranded DNA virus with a naked capsid and an average size of 20 nm. The infection has been called fifth disease in children and is usually mild with an incubation of 4–12 days. It manifests itself as exanthem infectiosum characterized by fever, headache, myalgia, malaise and itch with a confluent macular rash. The infection occurs most commonly in spring, and diagnosis is by DNA probes or ELISA.

## D. Poxviruses

Poxviruses are large double-stranded DNA viruses with a complex morphology. The poxvirus having human clinical significance has been smallpox, which historically had been one of the scourges of mankind. The smallpox viruses variola major and variola minor were fatal in 35% and 1% of those infected, respectively. Smallpox was ultimately eradicated in 1977 as the result of the successful implementation of a vaccine. Other poxviruses include (a) orf in sheep and goats, which cause a pustular dermatitis in farmers, (b) milkers' nodules, which occurs on the hands of milkers, (c) monkeypox and (d) cowpox. Serious concerns exist about the resurgence of smallpox as a weapon of bioterrorism. The vaccinia virus, a poxvirus, a variation of which serves as the vaccine against smallpox, is used commonly as a cloning vector with applications in molecular biology.

## XI. ARBOVIRUSES

A number of viruses are transmitted to humans through arthropod vectors (i.e. mainly insects) as well as animals. These types of viruses spread from humans only infrequently and almost invariably are spread through animals. These viruses overall can either produce mild disease or result in considerable mortality. However, many of these diseases are not frequently encountered in the U.S. The arboviruses are defined as arthropod-borne viruses, include over 400 species and are spread by mosquitoes, ticks and fleas. On the whole, the viruses are cytolytic and establish a systemic infection. The pathology is generally determined by the route of entry, the concentration and tropism. The diseases that arboviruses can induce include acute CNS disease including aseptic meningitis, encephalitis and encephalomyelitis, undifferentiated febrile illness with or without rash as well as hemorrhagic fevers. Examples of viral groups which include arboviruses are flaviviruses, alphaviruses, arenaviruses, bunyaviruses, reoviruses and filoviruses. Flaviviruses are single-stranded positive non-segmented enveloped viruses. They include the encephalitis viruses: St. Louis, Japanese, dengue. These usually produce mild systemic disease. However, in the case of dengue virus, exposure to a related strain of dengue after initial infection can result in severe hemorrhagic disease with associated shock, presumably through an antibody mediated enhancement of infection. Another example of a flavivirus is yellow fever, which can cause severe systemic disease with gastrointestinal hemorrhages and a mortality of up to 50%. Alphaviruses likewise are single-stranded positive nonsegmented enveloped viruses that can result in flu-like symptoms. Examples are the Venezuelan, Western and Eastern equine encephalitis viruses that can infect both humans and horses. Arenaviruses are single-stranded negative-polarity segmented enveloped viruses with a sandy appearance under the EM (from the Greek word *arenosa* meaning sandy). The viruses are zoonoses (i.e. spread by vertebrate animals) and include lymphocytic choriomeningitis virus (LCMV) and the hemorrhagic virus Lassa fever. Bunyaviruses are negative single-stranded RNA viruses with a segmented envelope. Examples of bunyaviruses include California encephalitis virus, which causes a febrile illness; Hantavirus, which can cause hemorrhagic renal or pulmonary manifestations; and Rift Valley fever (a phlebovirus), which causes a hemorrhagic fever. Colorado tick fever is an example of a reovirus. Filoviruses are non-enveloped negative-polarity single-stranded RNA viruses. The Ebola and Marburg viruses comprise the filovirus family. They are the most severe of the virally caused hemorrhagic fevers and are characterized by a very high morbidity and mortality.

## XII. RHABDOVIRUSES

Rhabdoviruses are bullet-shaped, enveloped, negative-stranded RNA viruses which replicate in the cytoplasm. Rabies virus is the pathogenic rhabdovirus in humans. It is usually transmitted through the bite of an infected animal in which the incubation period is related to the proximity of the site of infection to the CNS. During infection from several weeks to months, the virus infects the peripheral nerves and travels up the CNS to the brain. During the neurologic phase of infection, the classic symptoms, including hallucinations, tumors, delirium, hydrophobia and coma, occur, resulting invariably in death. A hallmark of the infection and disease is that an antibody response is not produced until late in the infection. Diagnosis of rabies is made serologically as well as neurocytopatho-logically for the presence of the diagnostic Negri bodies. Human rabies is very rare, but a large number of individuals receive rabies prophylaxis annually. Prophylaxis includes local treatment of the wound and instillation of anti-rabies antiserum around the wound. This is usually then followed by administration of a human diploid vaccine (HDCV) given on days 0, 3, 7, 14 and 28 days post-exposure. Pre-exposure vaccinations are usually given to animal handlers as well as veterinarians.

## XIII.  PERSISTENT VIRAL INFECTIONS OF THE CNS

A number of progressive neurological diseases are caused by viral or unconventional/unclassified agents. These diseases have also often been called slow viral diseases. The agents discussed can persistently infect neurons, macrophages, or lymphoid cells, and the resulting diseases are often fatal. The slow viruses include those belonging to the polyomaviruses. These are relatively ubiquitous viruses which usually do not cause disease. The infection is through the respiratory tract. Lymphocytes are the targets, and latency occurs in the kidneys. Immunosuppression causes reactivation and virus replication in the kidneys and the CNS. These diseases often occur in AIDS patients and others that are immunosuppressed. Examples of these viruses are the JC virus, which causes progressive multifocal leukoencephalopathy (PML), a subacute fatal demyelinating disease, as well as BK virus, which causes nephritis. Diagnosis is by histological methods, PCR or viral culture in the urine. No specific treatment or specific prevention exists for these agents. Chronic measles virus infection can also be characterized as a slow virus infection. It causes a condition known as subacute sclerosing panencephalitis (SSPE). The clinical symptoms of SSPE are insidious personality changes followed by blindness and spasticity, with death occurring within 6–12 months of the start of these symptoms. It usually occurs 2–10 years following infection with measles but occurs under the age of 20. It affects the gray and white matter of the brain, results in progressive dementia and neural degeneration and is invariably fatal. Unconventional "slow" viruses or agents include the prions, which are filterable agents that are typically resistant to formaldehyde, UV and heat. The prion represents a novel agent in that it does not contain nucleic acids; it therefore is an "infectious agent" devoid of any genetic material. The hypothesis is that the prions interact with normal host proteins and convert them into prions; these then aggregate as insoluble plaques that lead to progressive brain damage. Importantly, there is a lack of immune responses to prions. Overall, the disorders caused by prions are called transmissible spongiform encephalopathies (TSE). They are characterized by a progressive degeneration of neurons and axons with vacuolation of neurons. Specific TSEs are (a) kuru, which was transmitted through ritualistic cannibalism in New Guinea; (b) Creutzfeldt–Jakob disease (CJD), which can be transmitted through transplantation, contact with medical devices such as contaminated neurosurgical instruments and through a genetic defect in the prion protein (i.e. familial CJD); (c) scrapie, a disease of sheep; and (d) mad cow disease, which can occur in cows fed a "supplement" containing sheep brains. There is some suggestion and evidence that there is possible transmission to humans through eating contaminated beef. There is no treatment for the TSEs, and they are all invariably and progressively fatal.

## XIV.  DNA TUMOR VIRUSES

Several viral groups can be considered to be human DNA tumor viruses. These include (herpesviruses such as Epstein Barr virus), KSHV (Kaposi's sarcoma virus) as well as hepatitis B and the papillomaviruses. The criteria for indication that a DNA virus is a tumor virus are as follows: (a) a stable association of the viral genome with tumors, (b) the *in vitro* immortalization and oncogenic transformation of normal cells by the virus or genes, (c) expression of viral oncogenes in tumors as well as (d) epidemiological data. The herpesviruses (including the Kaposi's sarcoma viruses) and hepatitis B viruses have been described and summarized elsewhere in a subsection of this chapter.

## XV.  HUMAN PAPILLOMAVIRUSES (HPV)

HPVs belong to the papovaviruses and are double-stranded viruses with a circular DNA genome. They replicate in differentiating epithelium or mucosa, and latency can occur in the basal cell layer. Pathogenesis of HPVs involves infection of cells which induces cell proliferation. Activation of the E6 and E7 oncogenes occurs through disruption of the negative regulator E2 as a result of integration. The E6 oncoprotein forms a complex with the p53 tumor suppressor protein which inactivates p53 while the E7 oncoprotein complex inactivates the pRb105 retinoblastoma tumor suppressor. The cell cycle is then activated, and uncontrolled cell growth ensues. The major disease conditions associated with the HPVs include (a) skin warts (plantar, common and flat warts); (b) benign head and neck tumors (laryngeal, oral and conjunctival papillomas); (c) benign anogenital warts; and (d) cervical and penile malignancies. Development of cell mediated immunity is important against HPVs. Infection is through direct and sexual contact with the virus being relatively insensitive to inactivation. Diagnosis of infection includes hybridization of strain-specific DNA probes, PCR with strain-specific primers and the Papanicolaou (PAP) smears. A recently tested vaccination strategy against HPV has shown some potential efficacy for the prevention of cervical carcinoma due to HPV infection.

## XVI.  RETROVIRUSES

Retroviruses are enveloped viruses that contain two copies of single-stranded RNA of positive polarity. Following infection, the retroviral RNA genome is copied into single- and then double-stranded DNA by the viral enzyme reverse transcriptase, and this viral DNA then integrates into the host cell DNA. HIV-I and HIV-II are two important human retroviral pathogenic agents of acquired immune deficiency syndrome. The human T cell lymphotropic type I virus is an oncogenic retrovirus involved in adult T cell leukemia as well as a nonmalignant myelopathy syndrome.

Three subfamilies of retroviruses have been described: (a) the oncoviruses, with the human members including the human T cell lymphotropic (leukemia) viruses I and II (i.e. HTLV I and II); (b) the lentiviruses, with the human members including the human immunodeficiency viruses 1 and 2 (i.e. HIV 1 and 2); and (c) the spumaviruses, with the human members including the human foamy virus. The pathogenic human retroviruses are HTLV-I, HIV-1 and HIV-2. Oncoviruses are the only retroviruses that can immortalize or transform target cells. Lentiviruses can be characterized as clinically slow viruses that are associated with neurological and immunosuppressive disease. Spumaviruses (i.e. foamy viruses), as the name implies, cause a distinct cytopathologic effect but do not seem, currently, to cause human disease. Structurally, human retroviruses have three genes encoding polyproteins: gag (group specific antigen), pol (polymerase) and env (envelope). In the case of HTLV and HIV, regulatory genes are also present that control viral replication on the transcriptional level. These are rev and tat for HIV and rex and tax for HTLV.

A generalized diagrammatic representation of an HIV virion is given in Fig. 4-4. Infection and replication are initiated by the binding of the viral glycoprotein spikes (gp120 and gp41) to specific cell surface receptor proteins (i.e. CD4 and the secondary receptor, which have recently been identified as several chemokine receptors). After infection, the RNA genome is converted to double-stranded DNA, which integrates into the host genome. Virus (i.e. new) is then released from the infected cell by "budding" through the cell membrane containing the viral envelope proteins.

## A. Human Immunodeficiency Virus (HIV)

The major determinant in pathogenesis and disease caused by HIV is the viral tropism for CD4 expressing T cells and macrophages. The virion contains outer envelope proteins gp120 (attachment protein) and gp41 (membrane fusion), the matrix and capsid proteins and the reverse transcriptase, integrase and RNAse H (Fig. 4-4). In addition to the regulatory genes mentioned above, other gene products referred to as accessory genes are present: nef, vif, vpr and vpu.

The modes of Infection for HIV are sexual contact, contaminated blood (almost non-existent now, at least in developed industrialized countries) and vertical (i.e. mother to child) transmission. Neutralizing antibodies and cytotoxic T cells (CTL) are generated against HIV. However, because of viral escape mutants, these immunological mechanisms are ineffective in ultimately controlling infection and the development of AIDS. Laboratory diagnosis includes viral isolation from primary T cells and serum antibody detection by ELISA and Western blotting and by PCR (polymerase chain reaction). Treatment options for HIV include reverse transcriptase inhibitors such as zidovudine (AZT), dideoxyinosine (ddI) and dideoxycytidine (ddC), as well as the new protease inhibitors. "Triple" drug therapy has shown some promise. However, because of the nature

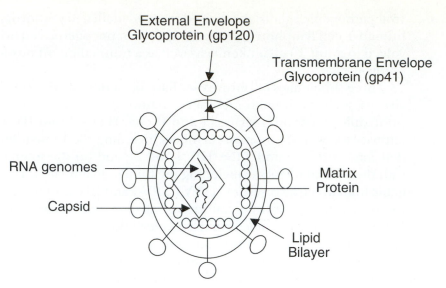

Figure 4-4.  Basic structure of HIV particle.

of the virus, the development of escape mutants have and will continue to result in the development of viral resistance, which will require the continued development and testing of new anti-retroviral agents. A number of experimental HIV vaccines as well as some currently in phase I, II and III trials are being aggressively tested. However, as with anti-retroviral therapy, the development of HIV escape mutants has seriously compromised the development of a vaccine against HIV. This is still a critically important area because it is acknowledged that the only way to control the HIV/AIDS pandemic is through an efficacious prophylactic vaccine.

## B. Human T Cell Leukemia (Lymphotropic) Viruses (HTLV I and II)

HTLV-I was the first human retrovirus described that was associated with human disease. It belongs to the oncovirus subfamily of retroviruses. It is the causal agent of adult T cell leukemia (ATL) and is strongly associated with HTLV-I associated myelopathy (HAM), which is also known as tropical spastic pareparesis (TSP). Endemic "pockets" of seropositivity exist is southwestern Japan, the Caribbean basin, the southeastern United States and parts of Africa. Worldwide total seropositivity is estimated to be 10–20 million. Serious disease manifestations of infection (i.e., ATL or HAM) develop in approximately 2–4% of those infected. The transcription activator, tax, can activate specific genes, i.e. IL-2 and IL-2 receptor α, which may be involved in the tumorigenicity of HTLV-I. The clinical latency between infection with HTLV-I and development of disease may be 30–50 years.

Transmission of HTLV infection is through sex and intravenous drug use as well as by breast feeding. Due to the long latency period between infection and development of ATL, transmission through breast feeding is thought to be important for the development of disease associated with HTLV-I infection. Cessation of breast feeding in Japan has significantly decreased the incidence of HTLV-I infection and hopefully will be effective in decreasing the incidence of ATL. Laboratory diagnosis of infection includes the same methods as used for HIV-I, i.e., ELISA and Western blotting as well as molecular techniques such as PCR.

Animal models (i.e. rats and rabbits) exist for HTLV-I infection and experimental vaccination of these species have resulted in protective immunity. However, no vaccine has been developed which has been demonstrated to be successful in humans. In terms of therapy, HTLV-I associated ATL has been shown to be recalcitrant to any treatment, and the disease has been shown to be invariably fatal within 6–12 months.

# Medical Mycology 5

*Susan Pross, PhD, and Sharon Hymes, MD*

## I. INTRODUCTION

The Kingdom Fungi is composed of nonphotosynthetic heterotrophs that rely on organic matter for their food. Fungi obtain their nutrients by acting either as decomposers, using dead animals and plants as their carbon source, or as parasites, getting their source of carbon from the living. Most fungi are obligate aerobes, requiring the presence of oxygen, with a few types of fungi being facultative anaerobes, thus growing well in more adverse environmental conditions. Of the greater than 80,000 species of fungi, most types are beneficial. They contribute to the foods we eat (examples include mushrooms and truffles, which are fungi, as well as bread, cheese and beer, which fungi help produce), the maintenance of our environment (degradation of waste products) and the health industry (production of antibiotics, including penicillin). Only a very small proportion of fungi are etiological agents of human disease, and these diseases range from being relatively harmless, resulting only in minor cosmetic manifestations, to causing significant morbidity and mortality when systemic involvement is present. The impact of a given fungal infection depends upon the interaction of that parasite and the host. This relationship, and the clinical manifestations of the infections, is contingent upon the genus and species of the fungus involved, as well as on the immune status of the individual. This section will review the basic structure and physiology of fungi and then concentrate on four groupings of fungal diseases: superficial/cutaneous, subcutaneous, systemic and opportunistic infections.

## II. FUNGAL STRUCTURE

In contrast to bacteria, which are prokaryotic, all fungi are eukaryotic. Their cells thus have membrane-bound nuclei, mitochondria, Golgi bodies, rough endoplasmic reticulum (ribosomes are bound) and cytoskeletons composed of microtubules and microfilaments. Fungi do not have endotoxins or bacterial-type exotoxins. The cell walls of fungi are composed primarily of complex carbohydrates, including chitin, in contrast to the peptidoglycans found in bacterial cell walls. This difference in cell wall structure between bacteria and fungi is medically significant because it renders fungi resilient to degradation by most microorganisms as well as creates resistance to the antibiotics used to inhibit bacteria, such as penicillin, whose action is to inhibit peptidoglycan synthesis. Although the membranes of fungi and of humans both contain cholesterol, the cell membranes of fungi contain both ergosterol and zymosterol. This is of medical significance, as the difference in membrane sterols renders the fungi sensitive to destructive by a variety of systemic agents.

## III. FUNGAL CYTOLOGY

Fungi are described as yeasts, molds or dimorphic organisms, depending on their growth and reproductive characteristics. Characteristically, yeasts grow as single cells and their method of reproduction is by budding. In contrast, molds grow as long filaments called hyphae. These filaments can group together, forming a mat-like structure called a mycelium. The hyphae can be further described as septate (in which there are transverse walls) or nonseptate (where the hyphae are multinucleated). Dimorphic fungi can exist either as yeasts or as molds, depending in part upon temperature. In this regard, many medically relevant fungi are thermally dimorphic and exist as molds in the cool environment and as yeast in the warm host.

## IV. FUNGAL REPRODUCTION

Reproduction in some fungi is characterized by the formation of sexual spores called zygospores (single, large), ascospores (formed in a sac, or ascus), and basidiospores (formed at the tip of a pedestal, or basidium) (see Fig. 5-1).

Other fungi, including most medically important fungi, do not form sexual spores, and they are classified as Fungi Imperfecti. These fungi reproduce by forming asexual spores called conidia, which branch off from specialized fungal structures. Examples of these types of asexual spores are arthrospores (fragmentation of hyphal ends), chlamydospores (round, thick-walled, resistant), blastospores (formed by budding) and sporangiospores (within a sac, or sporangium) (see Fig. 5-2). Specific

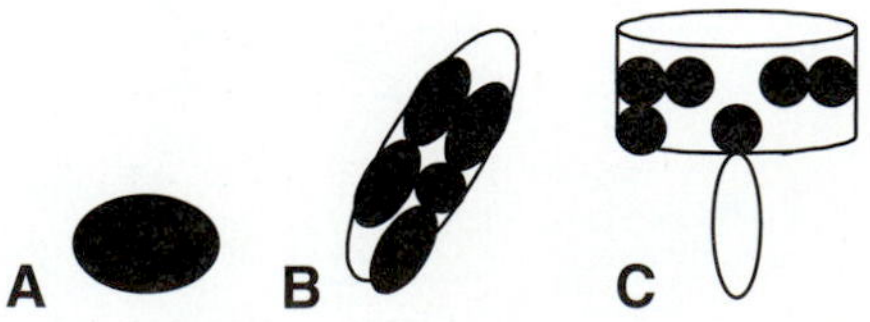

Figure 5-1. Sexual spores in fungi:
(**A**) zygospores; (**B**) ascospores;
(**C**) basidiospores.

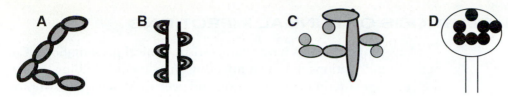

Figure 5-2. Asexual spores in fungi: (**A**) arthrospores; (**B**) chlamydospores; (**C**) blastospores; (**D**) sporangiospores.

characteristics of these conidia, including their shape and color, aid in the identification, and ultimately in the treatment, of the fungus.

## V. HOST–PARASITE INTERACTIONS

Fungi can impact on human health in three basic ways: by causing intoxications, by acting as allergens and by initiating an infectious process. Fungal intoxications, called mycotoxicoses, occur after ingesting a specific toxin from a pertinent fungus. Examples of such medically relevant intoxications may occur after eating *Amanita* mushrooms, which have a deadly hepatotoxin, consuming grain products contaminated with the mold *Claviceps purpura*, with alkaloids including ergotamine having potent vascular and neurological impacts, and ingesting grains and peanut products contaminated with *Aspergillus flavus*, whose aflatoxins result in liver damage. In addition, Type I hypersensitivities (IgE based) are characteristic of the reaction to certain types of fungal infections. Usually, the allergen is the fungal spore, and a medically relevant example is the reaction to the spores of *Aspergillus*, a fungus commonly found in the soil. The reaction is typical of other IgE allergies in that there is a wheal and flare to skin tests, and asthma may occur following antigenic exposure. In addition to inducing intoxication and allergy, fungal exposure can result in disease by an infectious process. Fungi gain entry into the body through a variety of approaches, including, in the case of superficial mycoses, transference from person to person, perhaps by sharing infected clothing, trauma, in which the skin is penetrated, often by a scratch from a piece of wood, and inhalation, in which the fungus enters the lungs, whereby an immunocompromised individual may have more difficulty handling this type of fungal exposure. In general, with the exception of some superficial infections, mycoses are not readily transmitted from patient to patient. Therefore, patients with fungal pneumonias are not normally isolated and hospital personnel are generally not required to wear masks and gowns. Effective protection against fungal infections includes various aspects of the innate immune system. The skin and mucous membranes create boundaries that protect the host from fungi in the environment. Fatty acids in the skin serve to inhibit fungal growth, as does the normal flora of both the skin and mucous membranes. In addition to these nonspecific protections against fungal infection, cellular immunity is also important in protection against fungi. In this regard, neutrophil killing, the action of macrophages and T cell immunity all are critical in terms of resistance to fungal disease.

## VI. DIAGNOSIS OF FUNGAL INFECTIONS

Many fungal diseases have characteristic clinical presentations. Cutaneous manifestations of fungal infections may include scaling, maceration, dyspigmentation, inflammation and pruritis. When these symptoms are present in a classic distribution, a presumptive diagnosis may be made. However, diagnostic tests and cultures are often performed to rule out bacterial infections or even neoplastic processes that present with similar clinical findings. Infections in immunocompromised patients may be atypical in morphology and location. Precise identification of genus and species of the fungus involved may be very important in such patients, requiring culture and sensitivity determinations. Some fungal organisms may fluoresce under a Wood's lamp—a source of ultraviolet light—aiding in their collection and identification. When laboratory diagnosis is needed, several approaches in terms of fungal identification are successful, including direct microscopic examination of the infected material, looking for spores, capsules and hyphae. The typical types of specimens used for fungal diagnoses may include hair, skin scrapings, sputum, CSF and lung biopsy material. The specimens are handled in a variety of ways, including the use of fungal stains that bind to fungal cell walls, the use of India ink to reveal capsules, and treatment of the specimens with solutions of 10% KOH in order to dissolve human cell walls, leaving the fungi intact. Culturing of specimens can be done at room temperature on special media such as Sabouraud's agar, which inhibits bacterial proliferation and optimizes growth of fungi. Culturing allows the use of DNA probes, currently available for only some fungi, for quick identification of the fungi in the early stages of growth, both in terms of genus and species, or, when time permits, visualization of characteristic mycelium and conidia. Systemic fungal infections can be diagnosed by serology, whereby antibody titers in serum or spinal fluid may be assessed.

## VII. TREATMENT OF FUNGAL INFECTIONS

Therapy for fungal infections ranges from surgical removal of infected areas to the use of systemic and topical antifungal agents. Older topical therapies, such as keratolytic agents, disrupt the stratum corneum and thereby interfere with the viability of superficial organisms. Selenium sulfide was found to interfere with both corneocytes and fungi, rendering it useful in both seborrheic dermatitis and tinea versicolor. Newer agents target physiological differences between the fungus and its host. Topical antifungal preparations of different classes are commonly used to treat a wide variety of cutaneous fungal infections. Benzofuranes (e.g., griseofulvin) inhibits fungal reproduction by blocking DNA synthesis, while benzimidazoles (e.g., ketoconazole) and triazoles (e.g., itraconazole, fluconazole) inhibit ergosterol syntheses in the fungal cell membrane. Allylamine derivatives (e.g., terbinafine) cause the accumulation of squalene, which blocks sterol synthesis. Systemic treatments often make use of drugs such as standard and liposomal amphotericin B, which acts by binding to ergosterol in the fungal membrane, forming channels and resulting in leaks, as well as the use fluconazole, ketoconazole and itraconazole.

Newer systemic antifungal agents, including the glucan synthesis inhibitor caspofungin, which inhibits the synthesis of $\beta$-(1,3)-D-glucan, an essential component of the cell wall of susceptible filamentous fungi, has also been helpful. The recent addition of broad spectrum triazole voriconazole may prove useful in the treatment of resistant fungal organisms, as it inhibits cytochrome P-450-mediated 14$\alpha$-lanosterol demethylation, essential in fugal ergosterol biosynthesis. In terms of the efficacy of these drugs for fungal treatment, it is important and challenging to correctly identify the fungus and to also minimize toxicity to the host.

## VIII. SUPERFICIAL AND CUTANEOUS MYCOSES

### A. General Comments

Superficial cutaneous mycoses (to be classified here as one group) represent fungal diseases characterized by their confinement either to the outer layers of the skin (stratum corneum) or to the nails and the hair. The limited niches of these fungi are due in part to various host factors including an intact skin surface, turnover of epithelial cells, ciliary action, fatty acids and environmental pH. External factors that disrupt the epidermal barrier, such as skin hydration or occlusion, may exacerbate these infections. Some of these mycoses cause predominantly cosmetic problems that are readily diagnosed and treated. Other fungi in this classification have more clinical significance, resulting in significant symptomatology or secondary bacterial infection.

Yeast infections may be predominately cutaneous, including pityriasis (tinea) versicolor, piedra, tinea nigra and candidiasis. Other fungal diseases with cutaneous involvement include those caused by dermatophytes. The pathology of these fungal infections relates to characteristics of the fungus as well as to the immune status of the host. For instance, the host may respond to a primary dermatophyte infection with a cellular immune response, termed an "id" (referring to dermatophytid) reaction. This reaction manifests as an eczematous eruption distant from the site of infection.

Dermatophytes may be divided according to genera, *Epidermophyton, Trichophyton* and *Microsporum,* which are differentiated from each other by sporulation patterns. Another approach is to categorize them by their clinical presentation. Occasionally it is useful to consider the source of the infection. Geophilic fungi may be found in the soil, while zoophilic fungi are transmitted by animals. Anthropophilic fungi are transmitted between humans. Diagnostic aids include a filtered ultraviolet light (Wood's light) that produces a characteristic fluorescence when shined on the affected body site, enabling the clinician to choose particular hairs or skin areas to examine for fungal hyphae and arthrospores. The scrapings may then be cultured at room temperature on Sabouraud's agar or dermatophyte test medium. Fungal identification is based both on resultant colonial morphology and microscopic characteristics. Treatment of these diseases ranges from the use of topical ointments and creams to oral therapy for more recalcitrant infections. The topical treatments are often needed for long periods of time and have limited successes, as with fungal disease of the nail. The primary oral antifungal drugs that treat both cutaneous yeast and dermatophyte infections are itraconazole, ketoconazole and fluconazole. Terbinafine and griseofulvin are useful in the treatment of dermatophyte infections.

## B. Specific Examples

### 1. Superficial Cutaneous Candidiasis

*Candida* species, most commonly *C. albicans,* are yeasts that may cause cutaneous infections in both healthy and immunosuppressed individuals. In terms of their cutaneous manifestations, interruption of the stratum corneum, either by maceration or trauma, may predispose the area to such infection. Due to their association with immunosuppressed patients, these diseases will be discussed in greater detail in the section on opportunistic infections.

### 2. Pityriasis (Tinea) Versicolor

a. **General Characteristics.** This superficial infection caused by *Malassezia furfur,* yeast, presents with scaly, macular lesions manifesting in areas rich in sebaceous glands, primarily on the upper torso, the arms, the legs and occasionally the abdomen. The fungus produces a chemical that interferes with melanin deposition, resulting in hypopigmented macules. Hyperpigmented lesions may be produced by thickened lesions containing the yeast. The differential pigmentation is accentuated after sun exposure, as affected areas will not tan.

b. **Clinical Issues and Diagnosis.** Diagnosis is confirmed by microscopic observation of skin scrapings, where hyphae and yeast are seen, leading to the descriptive terminology of "spaghetti and meatballs." Just as this fungus seeks out the fatty acids of sebaceous glands, the laboratory culturing requires special medium supplemented with fatty acids, and therefore it does not grow on Sabouraud's agar.

c. **Treatment.** Topical agents useful in this condition are selenium sulfide or imidazoles. Oral imidazoles are useful in extensive cases, but pityriasis versicolor does tend to recur.

### 3. Black Piedra

a. **General Characteristics.** This superficial asymptomatic infection is most common in Central and South America as well as in South East Asia. It usually presents on the scalp, but also in the beard, moustache and pubic areas, as hair displaying a hard and gritty texture. This grainy feel to the hair is due to the presence of nodules along the hair shaft. These nodules house the asci and ascospores (sexual phase) of the etiological agent of this disease, *Piedrai hortae,* an ascomycetous fungus.

b. **Clinical Issues and Diagnosis.** Diagnosis of this disease is made by clinical appearance, and confirmation is by direct microscopic examination of the hair. If hair samples are cultured on Sabouraud's agar, the asexual phase of the fungus will grow as dark colonies.

c. **Treatment.** Treatment of this disease is traditionally by either shaving or closely cropping the hair in order to remove the fungus and/or using oral and topical antifungal agents such as ketoconazole.

4. **White Piedra**

   a. **General Characteristics.** This rare superficial fungal infection, found most commonly in tropical and subtropical regions, presents as hair with white soft nodules due to a creamy deposit resultant to growth of the fungus *Trichosporon beigelii* on the outer part of the hair shaft. The white nodules are actually composed of mycelia, which fragment into arthrospores. The hair of the axilla or scalp is most commonly affected, and the major concern with this infection is cosmetic.

   b. **Clinical Issues and Diagnosis.** When the hair is treated with KOH, the hyphae are visualized. When hair samples are cultured on Sabouraud's agar, a dimorphic growth is noted: hyphae, arthroconidia and blastoconidia.

   c. **Treatment.** Treatment of this disease is traditionally by cutting or shaving the hair in order to physically remove the fungus, by the use of topical azoles or by systemically treating by the oral use of ketoconazol.

5. **Tinea Nigra**

   a. **General Characteristics.** This superficial infection is usually caused by *Exophiala werneckii*, a dimorphic fungus, and is characterized by brown to black macular lesions located primarily, but not exclusively, on the palms and soles. It is most commonly seen in tropical and subtropical environments where the etiological mold inhabits the soil.

   b. **Clinical Issues and Diagnosis.** The diagnosis is suggested by clinical presentation, but the presentation may be similar to that of melanoma or other melanocytic lesions, stains and general inflammation. Therefore, laboratory confirmation is often needed, and scrapings are acquired from the edges of scaly lesions. Microscopy of these scrapings will show darkly pigmented yeast-like cells and hyphal fragments.

   c. **Treatment.** Treatment is topical with either keratolytic agents or other antifungal creams and ointments.

6. **Dermatophytosis**

   a. **General Characteristics.** This grouping relates to infections caused by fungi of the genera *Trichophyton*, *Epidermophyton* and *Microsporum* that invade only the dead tissues of the skin or of its appendages. The zoophilic fungi, *Microsporum canis*, *Trichophyton mentagrophytes* and *Trichophyton verrucosum*, tend to cause significant inflammation, while the anthropophilic fungi may not elicit a marked immune response. The word tinea is often used, followed by the specific infected body site: capitus, corporis, etc.

   b. **Clinical Issues and Diagnosis.** The classic cutaneous manifestation of dermatophytes infection may be an annular scaling patch with a raised margin, leading to the common name "ringworm." The margin is often erythematous, denoting an inflammatory area, wherein the center of the patch is paler in color and less inflamed. The cutaneous and immunologic reactions elicited by these organisms may be fairly mild and difficult to eradicate, with frequent remissions and exacerbations. In some people, these infections may be acute, causing vesicles, pustules and secondary bacterial infection. Occasionally, fungus-free skin lesions may develop elsewhere on the body. These lesions, called "id" reactions, are thought to represent hypersensitivity to the fungus.

c. **Treatment.** Topical azoles are useful, and oral agents may be added for recalcitrant or widespread infection.

7. **Tinea Barbae**

a. **General Characteristics.** Although infections of the beard area are usually of bacterial origin, they may in fact be fungal, most often of the *Trichophyton* spp. Such mycotic infections are often termed ringworm of the beard or barber's itch.

b. **Clinical Issues and Diagnosis.** The lesions of these fungal infections vary from mild, with diffuse erythema, to inflammatory, with pustules and scarring resulting in permanent hair loss.

c. **Treatment.** Although there may be some response to topical antifungal agents, oral agents are often necessary to eradicate the infection. Occasionally, a short course of prednisone is used in inflammatory cases, to minimize scarring and preserve the follicular unit.

8. **Tinea Capitus**

a. **General Characteristics.** These are fungal (*Trichophyton* spp., *Microsporum* spp.) infections of the scalp, eyebrows and eyelashes that occur most commonly in children before puberty, although they can occur in the elderly. This age demarcation is thought to relate to physiologic skin changes.

b. **Clinical Issues and Diagnosis.** In these infections, the fungus may invade the scalp as well as the hair shafts and follicles. The scalp develops crusts, and the hair may be shed late into the disease. The fungus can be passed from person to person, often through sharing of caps or hair brushes, and, in some cases, the fungus can be passed from an animal to a person, such as from a pet cat or dog. Tinea capitus may be relatively non-inflammatory, making it difficult to differentiate from dermatitis without a fungal culture. Wood's lamp evaluation is helpful only if a bright green fluorescence is seen in the affected areas, usually associated with *Microsporum* species. The most common pathogen, *T. tonsurans,* does not fluoresce. Occasionally a localized, well-demarcated, indurated area studded with vesicles and pustules, called a kerion, will develop, potentially resulting in scarring and permanent alopecia.

c. **Treatment.** Tinea capitus should be treated with systemic antifungal agents. In children, griseofulvin has been the mainstay of therapy, but fluconazole, itraconazole and terbinafine are proving to be very effective.

9. **Tinea Corporis**

a. **General Characteristics.** Often referred to as "ringworm" because of its annular morphology, this fungal disease, usually caused by *Trichophyton* spp., is primarily seen on the trunk and legs of infected individuals and is most common in tropical regions.

b. **Clinical Issues and Diagnosis.** The lesions may be pruritic, and the degree of inflammation varies depending on the specific etiological agent as well as the host. The clinical picture may resemble psoriasis or dermatitis, and identification of the fungus by microscopy and laboratory culture of skin scrapings may be necessary for accurate diagnosis of the clinical presentation.

c. **Treatment.** If localized, tinea corporis will respond to topical agents. Widespread lesions are better treated with oral fluconazole, itraconazole or terbinafine. Eradication of cutaneous fungal reservoirs, such as infected nails, may help prevent recurrences.

### 10. Tinea Cruris

a. **General Characteristics.** This fungal infection, commonly called "jock itch," is characterized by erythematosus, pruritic and scaly lesions in the groin, inner thighs and pubic or gluteal areas.

b. **Clinical Issues and Diagnosis.** It is typically found in young men, especially in macerated or occluded areas. It is often associated with tinea pedis (athlete's foot), and the causative organism may easily be seen in skin scrapings by KOH examination.

c. **Treatment.** Treatment is similar to that of tinea corporis. Minimizing the occlusive environment may encourage lasting remissions of this chronic infection.

### 11. Tinea Pedis

a. **General Characteristics.** These infections, often known as "athlete's foot," are caused most commonly by *Trichophyton rubrum* or *Trichophyton mentagrophytes*. This is a fairly common affliction, affecting immunocompetent individuals as well as people with depressed T cell function.

b. **Clinical Issues and Diagnosis.** The affected areas may be itchy and macerated, with scaling and blistering. Occasionally, the fungus will infect both feet and one hand, commonly called one-hand, two-feet disease. Once the integrity of the epidermis is breached, secondary bacterial infection may produce a cellulitis. The fungus can spread to other areas of the body, particularly to the toenails, resulting in onychomycosis.

c. **Treatment.** Chronic treatment with topical agents may minimize disease recurrence. Acute infections, especially with clinical vesiculation, and nail involvement respond best to oral agents such as itraconazole or terbinafine.

## IX. SUBCUTANEOUS MYCOSES

### A. General Comments

These relatively rare infections result from entry of fungi into the dermis, the subcutaneous tissue and even the bones of the individual. The etiological agents of these infections are predominantly from the environment, usually from the soil and decaying vegetation. They generally enter the body via a traumatic event, including scratches and punctures by plant stems and tree branches, and these fungi affect people with normal immune status. These infections are often challenging to diagnose, as they may resemble some bacterial infections, particularly of the genera *Staphylococcus, Nocardia* and *Actinomyces.* In addition, these infections tend to be difficult to treat, requiring systemic antifungal agents and possible surgical excision.

## B. Specific Examples

### 1. Lymphocutaneous Sporotrichosis

a. **General Characteristics.** This disease is commonly known as "gardener's disease" and is the most common of the subcutaneous fungal infections. The etiological agent is *Sporothrix schenckii*, a dimorphic fungus. In the body, *S. schenckii* grows as yeast, but on Sabouraud's agar at room temperature, characteristic hyphae that change from white to brown are noted, with a growth pattern referred to as a "rosette." The hyphal form converts to yeast at 37°C.

b. **Clinical Issues and Diagnosis.** Typically, an individual has worked in the yard or garden, especially with roses, and has been scratched, for instance, by a thorn contaminated with this fungus. The infected individual may first notice a small painless lesion at the inoculation site. The lesion then develops, becoming nodular, painful and ulcerative, moving along the lymphatics, away from the site of puncture.

c. **Treatment.** The treatment of choice is itraconazole, although a saturated solution of potassium iodide is also effective. Although the infection rarely progresses systemically, amphotericin B is recommended for those complications.

### 2. Chromoblastomycosis (Chromomycosis)

a. **General Characteristics.** This disease, rare in the United States, is characterized by lesions that have a verrucous (warty) appearance. Copper-colored spherical yeasts (Medlar bodies) can be identified in the tissue and help with the diagnosis. The etiological agents include several genera of a collection of soil fungi called dematiaceous fungi, a term used to denote the dark-brown to black pigments found in the fungal cell walls. The most common etiologic agent of this disease is *Fonsecaea pedrosoi*, but other species as well as genera including *Cladosporium* and *Phialophora* are also included in the diagnosis.

b. **Clinical Issues and Diagnosis.** The lesions of chromoblastomycosis initially appear at the site of fungal inoculation, and if the fungus is untreated, the lesions become verrucous and slowly spread. Laboratory diagnosis includes the visualization of characteristic thick-walled brown sclerotic cells on microscopy as well as characteristic fungal colonies on media.

   c. **Treatment.**  Treatment is usually prolonged with oral therapy in-
      cluding the use of itraconazole and fluconazole

3. **Phaeohyphomycosis**

   a. **General Characteristics.**  This term is used for a rare group of
      diseases, with similar albeit less intense clinical manifestations than
      chromoblastomycosis.

   b. **Clinical Issues and Diagnosis.**  The diseases are often charac-
      terized by the formation of subcutaneous cysts at the site of implan-
      tation of the fungus, and the cysts eventually become necrotic. The
      progress of the disease tends to be by expansion by satellite colonies,
      and the disease may demonstrate chronic to systemic manifestations.
      Just as with chromoblastomycosis, the etiological agents also belong
      to the general classification of dematiaceous fungi and are caused
      by a variety of genera within this descriptive group.

   c. **Treatment.**  Treatment options for phaeohyphomycosis include
      both surgery and chemotherapy. However, surgical resection is not
      always feasible. Amphotericin B, ketoconazole and miconazole have
      been used with only a modicum of success, but recent reports of the
      use of itraconazole have been more encouraging.

4. **Eumycotic Mycetoma**

   a. **General Characteristics.**  The term mycetoma, also termed
      madura foot, refers to infections that start out as a local infection in
      the subcutaneous tissue but undergo slow progressive spread through-
      out the subcutaneous tissue into the connective tissue and the bone.
      The etiological agents of eumycotic mycetomas, those caused by fungi,
      include members of the genera *Pseudallescheria* and *Madurella*. Eumy-
      cotic mycetomas are found primarily in tropical areas and are most
      common in India, Mexico, Saudi Arabia, Yemen and sub-Sahara
      Africa. The etiological fungi can be identified in the soil of the United
      States, but disease here is rare.

   b. **Clinical Issues and Diagnosis.**  These infections do not gener-
      ally become systemic. The disease manifests as indolent swollen lesions
      with draining into sinus tracts. The infection may initially be painless,
      but the resultant pathology is destructive, as the lesions grow and rup-
      ture. These manifestations can also be caused by bacteria, including
      members of the genera *Nocardia, Streptomyces* and *Actinomyces*. Fungal
      mycetomas are found primarily in young adult men, as they are usu-
      ally the individuals laboring in rural areas, thus exposing themselves
      to scratches and cuts by thorns and pieces of wood, allowing entry of
      the fungi into the subcutaneous tissue.

   c. **Treatment.**  Although the physical presentation is similar in myce-
      tomas of bacterial and fungal etiologies, the drugs of treatment are
      significantly different, and proper diagnosis is critical for successful
      treatment and recovery. Treatment includes surgical excision of the
      infected areas as well as medical approaches, including long-term
      treatment with diaminodiphenylsulfone or ketoconazol, depending
      on the specific fungus.

## X. SYSTEMIC INFECTION

### A. General

The fungi traditionally classified in this group are inherently virulent. This means that these agents cause disease in healthy people as well as in the immunosuppressed. Importantly, the characteristics of the disease still vary in relation to the immune status of the host.

### B. Specific Examples

#### 1. Histoplasmosis

a. **General Characteristics.** This disease is also known as Darling's disease, after the physician who described it, as well as cave disease and spelunker's disease, after the areas where it is most prevalent and the activities resulting in greatest risk. It is relatively common in the Midwest of the United States, around the Ohio and Mississippi Valley region, affecting around 500,000 people, and it has a worldwide distribution. It is caused when an individual inhales either the conidia or hyphal fragment of *Histoplasma capsulatum,* a dimorphic fungus that grows in soil with high nitrogen content. As such, it is present in large numbers in areas contaminated with bat and bird dropping (starlings and chickens). Although bats can be infected with *H. capsulatum,* birds are not.

b. **Clinical Issues and Diagnosis.** The clinical disease centers on the pulmonary system. Once either the conidia or the hyphal fragments are inhaled, they are phagocytized by pulmonary macrophages. The mold form then converts to yeast, which multiply within the macrophage, which contains the infection (see Fig. 5-3). Most immunocompetent people are asymptomatic, and the only evidence that they had been infected is based on serum titers and on unrelated autopsies where granulomas containing *H. capsulatum* can be seen. It is estimated that 5% of *H. capsulatum* infections result in a flu-like illness that tends to be acute and self-limited. The illness rarely needs to be treated in the immunocompetent host. In the immuno-

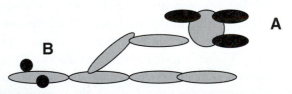

Characteristic Spores—Tuberculate macroconidia (**A**) and microconidia (**B**)

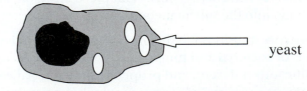

Macrophage with yeast phase of *H. capsulatum* in cytoplasm

Figure 5-3. *Histoplasma capsulatum*—spores (**top**) and yeast form (**bottom**).

compromised host, this infection can be problematic in that the yeast may not be contained in the lungs and the disease will disseminate and include CNS involvement.

Diagnosis of histoplasmosis is often not performed because of the relatively innocuous findings in most people. When it is reported, the diagnosis is based on serology, complement-fixation test, histopathology and antibody titer of infected tissue as well as culture characteristics. The mold form of *H. capsulatum* has distinct morphological characteristics, including delicate septate hyphae with tuberculate macroconidia that aid in identification. Recent tests include the use of an exoantigen test as well as DNA probes.

c. **Treatment.** Although most cases of histoplasmosis do not have to be treated, oral itraconazole and/or amphotericin B may be used for disseminated disease. Immunosuppressed patients need long-term treatment due to the high percent of cases that relapse.

## 2. Blastomycosis

a. **General Characteristics.** This systemic disease, caused by *Blastomyces dermatitidis*, is also known as Gilchrist's disease, after the physician who described it, or Chicago disease and North American blastomycosis, after the areas of highest prevalence. This disease, less common than histoplasmosis, is endemic in the Ohio and Mississippi Valley regions, overlapping in part with the situation with histoplasmosis as well as in Missouri, Arkansas, Minnesota and Southern Canada and in Northern Africa. Unlike histoplasmosis, the natural reservoir for this dimorphic fungus is not known as it is extremely difficult to find in the soil from endemic areas. In addition, blastomycosis is a significant problem in animals, specifically dogs and horses, in endemic areas.

Similar to the situation with histoplasmosis, blastomycosis is initiated by inhalation of conidia, body temperature initiates the conversion to the yeast phase, the yeast are phagocytized by pulmonary macrophages and the disease may be asymptomatic with successful resolution or can become systemic.

b. **Clinical Issues and Diagnosis.** This disease often is undiagnosed due to its vague symptoms and prompt resolution. However, in patients presenting to the physician with characteristic pulmonary symptoms, laboratory diagnosis may be warranted. In these cases, samples of infected tissue, often obtained from abscess fluid, are acquired and examined by microscopy where the characteristic broad-based yeast can be seen (see Fig. 5-4). The fungus converts to the mold phase in culture, displaying microconidia 2–4 μm long. Similar to histoplasmosis, an exoantigen test can also be utilized.

c. **Treatment.** Although most cases of this disease resolve without treatment, itraconazole or fluconazole may be used for pulmonary manifestations, and amphotericin B may be needed in disseminated cases.

## 3. Paracoccidiomycosis

a. **General Characteristics.** This disease is often called South American blastomycosis after its major endemic area and is caused by *Paracoccidiodes brasiliensis,* a dimorphic fungus.

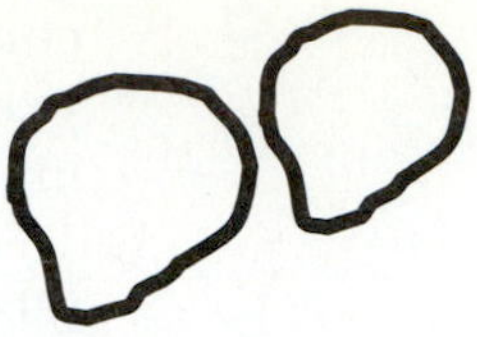

Figure 5-4. *Blastomyces dermatitides*—yeast form. Note the characteristic broad base of the yeast form.

    b. **Clinical Issues and Diagnosis.** Similar to *B. dermatitis*, the fungus is rarely isolated from the soil, and in most cases clinical disease is not apparent. The disease is usually diagnosed after dissemination to the buccal and nasal mucosa by visualization of the multipolar budding characteristics of the yeast, creating a characteristic hip's wheel pattern (see Fig. 5-5).

    c. **Treatment.** Treatment of paracoccidiomycosis is long-term therapy with amphotericin B as well as with azole drugs, including itraconazole and ketoconazole.

**4. Coccidioidomycosis**

    a. **General Characteristics.** This disease, caused by *Coccidioides immitis,* is commonly called Posadas–Wernicke disease, as well as San Joaquin Valley fever, and desert rheumatism after its epidemiological niches. It is found primarily in the Americas: North, Central and South. In the U.S., it is endemic in arid regions, including parts of California and Texas. Similar to histoplasmosis, the mold form can be readily isolated from the soil. Because *C. immitis* thrives in dry arid soil, it can be moved long distances by dust storms.

    b. **Clinical Issues and Diagnosis.** Unlike the relatively vague pulmonary presentations of the systemic fungal diseases discussed above, with some patients being asymptomatic and the rest having mild symptoms, coccidiomycosis often presents with symptoms that will range from a mild fever to a more serious respiratory disease. A small percent of people with this disease will develop meningitis and dermatological manifestations. Diagnosis is usually made by noting a characteristic growth (spherule, see Fig. 5-6) in sections of infected tissues. Skin test reactivity to antigens of the spherule phase or the mycelial phase may also be helpful. Serologic and immunologic tests are also helpful. *C. immitis* grows well in the laboratory, and a presumptive diagnosis can often be made. Culturing can be problematic for two reasons. *C. immitis* mold, due to its dispersive ability, can easily can contaminate a laboratory, and, in addition, the mold phase, although suggestive of *C. immitis,* is not determinative.

    c. **Treatment.** As with the previously discussed fungal infection, amphotericin B is the drug of choice and is fairly successful with the respiratory aspects of the infection, but results are not as impressive

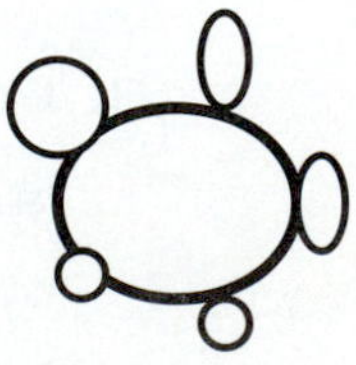

Figure 5-5. *Paracoccidioides brasiliensis*—yeast form. Note the multiple buds of the yeast phase.

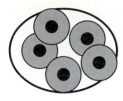

Figure 5-6. *Coccidioides immitis*—endospores. Note the spherule containing endospores, characteristic of *C. immitis*. The spherule forms after arthrospores differentiate within the body. When the spherule ruptures, the endospores are released, disseminate and form new spherules.

with the meningitis aspects. The specificity of the mold can be determined by the use of specific exoantigen tests.

## XI. OPPORTUNISTIC MYCOSES

### A. General Comments

Whereas the fungi discussed previously caused systemic disease in immunocompetent and immunocompromised individuals, the examples discussed in this section are not considered to be very pathogenic in immunocompetent individuals; however, there fungi are highly pathogenic in the immunocompromised. Therefore, fungi that exist in the environment can cause devastating diseases in people undergoing treatment for cancer, for transplant recipients, for people with AIDS or other illnesses, particularly where there is neutropenia. People who are very old or very young have more problems with fungal infections. Many of these fungal infections are associated with disease of the pulmonary and neurological systems. However, they also often have cutaneous manifestations, and their presentations in the immunocompromised can be complex. For example, a leukemic patient may present with an ulcerative cutaneous plaque that is in fact due, for example, to *Aspergillus*.

### B. Specific Examples

#### 1. Aspergillosis

a. **General Characteristics.** This disease can affect both healthy and immunocompromised people, but the manifestations are much more profound in the immunocompromised. The etiological agent is *Aspergillus* spp. (*A. fumigatus*, *A. flavus* and *A. niger*), a mold that can cause allergic manifestations as well as invasive disease. *A. fumigatus* (see Fig. 5-7) is a common cause of human disease, and it is found worldwide. It is ubiquitous and readily isolated from damp basements and from vegetation. Transmission is by inhalation of conidia, and this is particularly problematic in the immunocompromised patient. Therefore, construction areas near hospitals, where land is moved around, can be an important source of infection in resident neutropenic patients.

b. **Clinical Issues and Diagnosis.** The disease is characterized by blood vessel thrombosis and infarction as well as by blockage of airways from fungal masses. Aspergilloma refers to the formations of fungal

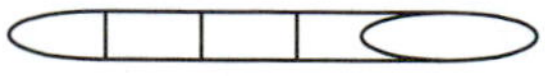

Figure 5-7. *Aspergillus fumigatus*. Note the septate hyphae, characteristic of *A. fumigatus*.

balls within infected lungs or sinus cavities. In addition, allergic reactions to this fungus result in asthmatic types of conditions. Laboratory diagnosis is fairly easy because *A. fumigatus* grows well on laboratory media, resulting in small, fluffy white colonies as well as characteristic sporulation within 2 days.

c. **Treatment.** Treatment of this disease is usually with systemic amphotericin B or itraconazole. Voriconazole and caspofungin are newer systemic antifungal agents that have proven useful in the treatment of refractory invasive aspergillosis. In some cases, surgery may be required.

2. **Candidiasis**

a. **General Characteristics.** This disease has many forms—cutaneous and systemic—both caused most commonly by *Candida albicans,* a dimorphic fungus that exists as yeast on mucosal surfaces where it is a part of the normal flora, and thus a commensal, and forms hyphae when it is invasive.

b. **Clinical Issues and Diagnosis.** It is found in the skin, mouth and intestines of healthy individuals. Oral candidiasis, also called thrush, is characterized by creamy white patches on the tongue as well as on other areas of the oral mucosa. The patches are composed of the fungus, epithelial cells and leukocytes. The diagnosis is made by clinical impression and confirmed by scraping the material and searching for both the yeast and hyphal forms (see Fig. 5-8) by light microscopy. Resistance to *Candida* requires intact skin and mucosa. Maceration of the integument will allow entry of this organism and possible infections, even in healthy people. The clinical manifestations are variable and dependent on the anatomical site involved. For example, in intertriginous areas, *Candida* often manifests as indurated red plaques with satellite pustules. *Candida paronychia* presents with inflammation and even purulence at the nail folds, which must be differentiated from a bacterial infection. Infants may develop cutaneous candidiasis from direct maternal contact through a colonized birth canal. Alterations of normal bacterial flora with antibiotics, as well as hormonal therapy, pregnancy and diabetes, will encourage *Candida* colonization and infection. Immunocompetent individuals usually do not experience sepsis from *Candida*. Neutrophils primarily, but also lymphocytes, monocytes and even eosinophils are thought to contribute to the defense. Individuals who are neutropenic, or who have normal numbers of neutrophils but diminished myeloperoxidase, hydrogen peroxide or superoxide anion systems will have trouble containing these infections. In addition, the complement system, particularly the alter-

Figure 5-8. *Candida albicans*—endospores. Note the pseudohyphae (**A**) and budding yeast (blastospores) (**B**), characteristic of *C. albicans*. In the body, germ tubes (**C**) form, which are the beginning of true hyphae.

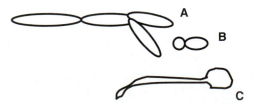

native pathway, is also thought to provide an important line of defense. Factors that impede the normal immune protective strategies of the host also lead to an increase in *Candida* infections. Diabetics tend to have more cutaneous infections, and these infections tend to be more extensive and difficult to eradicate. Iatrogenic infections occur in the setting of increased instrumentation of patients, including the use of catheters and respirators, and these procedures increase the risk of septicemia. When the organism infects visceral tissue, micro-abscesses are seen, containing both the yeast and hyphal forms and resulting in a granulomatous type of reaction. The people who are most susceptible to invasive candidiasis are those who are stressed, immunosuppressed and treated with antibiotics. Antibiotics create an imbalance between normal bacterial flora, allowing *Candida* proliferation. The result of such infections range from localized mucocutaneous lesions to significant invasions of all major organs.

c. **Treatment.** Treatment parameters are influenced by the immunologic status of the host. Many immunocompetent patients may be treated by topical azoles or even nystatin. Such patients often spontaneously clear their infection when the inciting factor (antibiotics, maceration, etc.) is corrected. Extensive infections should prompt the clinician to search for predisposing causes, including immunosuppression. Treatment may include systemic agents, such as fluconazole or itraconazole. Amphotericin or caspofungin may play a role in treating systemic disease.

## 3. Cryptococcosis

a. **General Characteristics.** This disease, caused by *Cryptococcus neoformans*, is also called Busse–Buschke disease, torulosis, or European blastomycosis, after its traditional environmental niche, but it really now has a worldwide distribution. Similar to *H. capsulatum*, *C. neoformans* is found in bird droppings. The relevant bird is the pigeon, which itself is not usually infected, but the fungus likes the high nitrogen content of the droppings. The fungus survives in a desiccated, alkaline, nitrogen-rich environment. Unlike all of the previous systemic fungi discussed above, the asexual stage of *C. neoformans* is a monomorphic fungus existing as yeast in the environment as well as in the body. This yeast is heavily encapsulated with polysaccharides, which serve to protect it from phagocytosis. This protection by the acidic mucopolysaccharide capsule of the fungus, along with potent virulence factors, make this a problematic fungus, especially in patients with impaired immunity. For example, AIDS patients have about a 10% chance of developing cryptococcal meningitis, higher than the incidence in people with healthy immune systems.

b. **Clinical Issues and Diagnosis.** There is a large range of clinical manifestations of this disease. Often times it is asymptomatic, but when symptomatic, the person may develop pneumonia or, more seriously, meningitis. *Cryptococcus* meningitis, caused by the spread of yeast from the lungs to the brain, is the most frequently diagnosed form of cryptococcal disease.

The yeast of *C. neoformans* has a very distinct appearance, making diagnosis of this infection clear when the cells are visualized. For example, India ink preparations of CSF of a patient with *Cryptococcus* meningitis may show a single cell of budding yeast surrounded by a clear halo due to the capsule excluding the ink (see Fig. 5-9). Isolation of the yeast is not possible in all cases of disease, and diagnosis then relies upon serology and culture.

c. **Treatment.** Cases of pulmonary cryptococcosis are usually asymptomatic and self-limited. When a pulmonary nodule is discovered, surgical excision is usually curative. If the disease disseminates, which occurs more commonly in immunocompromised hosts, the fatality rate approaches 100% since amphotericin B, active against *C. neoformans* in culture and in the lungs, has poor CNS penetration. Treatment with 5-fluorocytosine is often attempted because it has good CNS penetration, but it is not as effective against the fungus. Another approach to treatment, which has some success, is the use of a combination of drug therapy. Even with treatment with a combination of amphotericin B and 5-fluorocytosine, survival is <50% in AIDS patients. In addition, patients with AIDS generally will require lifelong antifungal treatment.

4. **Pneumocystosis**

a. **General Characteristics.** This disease is caused by *Pneumocystis carinii*, previously classified as a sporozoan protozoon but now considered to be a fungus. *P. carinii* is carried by many hosts as well as humans. Multiple organs can be affected, including the lungs, eyes, ears, liver, bone marrow and lungs. The organism can be identified by histology, and appropriate specimens include sputum and bronchoalveolar lavage. *P. carinii* can be transmitted from person to person by droplet inhalation, and thus close contact results in a higher chance of spread. Infection with this organism usually causes no clinical problem in healthy people but results in a pneumonia-like condition (PCP) that is severe in premature infants as well as in people who are immunocompromised, such as those who are elderly, malnourished or with AIDS.

b. **Clinical Issues and Diagnosis.** Pneumocystosis may start out as a mild fever and weakness, develop into interstitial pneumonitis, severe dyspnea and tachypnea and then result in death by asphyxiation. Radiographic studies of the lung reveal a characteristic "ground glass" look as the pulmonary infiltrates spread.

c. **Treatment.** The treatment of choice for pneumocystosis is trimethoprim-sulfamethoxazole used in combination with sulfamethoxazole or pentamidine, often in combination with supportive therapy.

5. **Zygomycosis**

a. **General Characteristics.** These diseases are very rare in healthy individuals but of significant clinical importance in debilitated

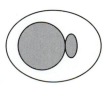

Figure 5-9. *Cryptococcus neoformans*—endospores. Note the characteristic wide capsule of *C. neoformans* visualized in an India ink stain.

patients, often leading to death. Zygomycosis is found in diabetics, malnourished individuals, burn patients, cancer patients and people with AIDS.

b. **Clinical Issues and Diagnosis.** The fungi (family *Mucorales* or *Entomophthorales*) tend to invade blood vessels and lead to the formation of emboli. The resultant areas of necrosis provide opportunity for fulminant bacterial growth. Areas typically affected include the rhino-facial-cranial regions as well as the lungs and the GI tract.

c. **Treatment.** Treatment is often with amphotericin B, but the course of this disease is rapid and fatalities are common.

# Medical Parasitology 6

*William Yotis, PhD, and Nicholas Legakis, MD*

## I. INTRODUCTION

The parasites are divided into the unicellular protozoa and the multicellular Metazoa helminths, both of which contain some organisms that are pathogenic for humans. The names of the four classes of protozoa are as follows: (1) Sporozoa—The organisms in this class undergo sporulation at some stage in the life cycle and are generally non-motile. The most important genus is *Plasmodium,* which causes malaria. (2) Mastigophora—This class includes basically the flagellated protozoa. Medically important genera are *Trepanosoma* and *Leishmania,* which cause sleeping sickness and leishmaniasis, respectively. (3) Sarcodina—These protozoa move and ingest food by means of pseudopodia. They have no definite morphology. *Endamoeba histolytica* is the most important pathogenic species that causes amebic dysentery. (4) Ciliates—This class characterized by cilia includes only one species, *Balantidium coli,* which produces a rare infection of the large intestine.

The Metazoa helminths, or worms, fall into two phyla: Platyhelminthes, or flatworms, including the trematodes (flukes) and cestodes (tapeworms); and Nemahelminthes, or threadworms, which are also called nematodes, or round worms.

Protozoa range in size from 2 to more than 100 μm. They contain a membrane-bound nucleus with a central nucleolus and cytoplasm. The cytoplasm contains an inner endoplasm and an outer thin ectoplasm, which is organized into specialized organelles of locomotion. In some protozoa these organelles are called pseudopodia; in others, cilia or flagella arise from intracytoplasmic granules. Most pathogenic protozoa are facultative anaerobes. They are also heterotrophic organisms that engulf soluble or particulate matter in digestive vacuoles by pinocytosis and phagocytosis.

The helminths or worms are elongated, bilaterally symmetric organisms which vary in length from less than a millimeter to more than 1 meter. The body is covered with an a tough cuticle. Helminths have primitive nervous and excretory systems and highly developed reproductive systems, and some have digestive tracts. Nemahelminthes have a cylindrical body with a tubular alimentary tract that extends from the mouth to the anus and exist as male and female roundworms. Platyhelminthes have ribbon-shaped bodies. The head or scolex of the tapeworms has suckers with hookers. Behind the head is a chain of reproductive segments called proglottids, each segment of which contains both male and female gonads. Tapeworms lack digestive tracts and absorb nutrients through the cuticle. Flukes are leaf-shaped worms with blind, branched digestive tracts. Two suckers, one on the mouth and one on the ventral site of the body, serve as organs of attachment and locomotion. Most flukes are hermaphroditic.

## II. ERYTHROCYTIC PROTOZOA

### A. *Plasmodium vivax, P. ovale, P. malariae, P. falciparum*

#### 1. Transmission and Life Cycle

Malaria, caused by the four species of plasmodia, is transmitted to humans by bites of the female *Anopheles* mosquitoes, and it is the most important parasitic disease. It affects more than 200 million annually persons in tropical communities and causes between 1 and 3 million deaths per year, almost all of which are due to *P. falciparum*.

The life cycle of the malaria parasites consists of the sexual phase, or sporogony, which occurs in the intermediate host, that is, the female anopheline mosquito, and the asexual phase, or schizogony, that occurs in an individual, which is the definitive host. During the sporogony, gametocytes in the gut of the female anopheline mosquito first form zygotes, then ookinetes, oocysts and finally infective sporozoites, which migrate to the salivary glands of the mosquito. Schizogony begins when an infected female mosquito bites an individual and injects sporozoites in his bloodstream. During the exoerythrocytic, or hepatic, cycle, the sporozoites infect liver cells and develop into schizonts, which release merozoites into the bloodstream.

Merozoites infect red blood cells and become trophozoites; these form schizonts and release more merozoites. Some merozoites that infect red blood cells become male and female gametocytes. The gametocytes are ingested by a female *Anopheles* mosquito when it bites a person infected with the plasmodium parasite.

#### 2. Pathogenesis and Clinical Manifestations

The hallmark of malaria is fever, which might be the result of the release of interleukin-1 (IL-1) and/or tumor necrosis factor (TNF) from macrophages involved in the ingestion of plasmodial or erythrocytic debris. Elevated IL-1 and TNF levels are consistently found in malaria. In untreated infections, *P. vivax* or *P. ovale* causes benign tertian malaria (fever of about 40°C every 2 days), *P. falciparum* produces malignant tertian malaria (fever over 40°C every 2 days), and *P. malariae* causes quartan malaria (fever every 3 days). The clinical symptoms vary with the species of plasmodia but generally include fever, chills, splenomegaly and anemia. After an incubation period of about 2 weeks, the patient has continuous rigors, feels cold, develops a temperature of 40–41.7°C (104–107°F) and then becomes afebrile. The decrease in body temperature ushers in profuse sweating. The symptoms cease when *Plasmodia* disappear from blood. Malaria caused by *P. falciparum* is more severe than that produced by other plasmodia because it is associated with high levels of parasitemia, infects red blood cells of all ages and occludes capillaries with aggregates of parasitized red blood cells, which leads to hemorrhages and necrosis. When the central nervous system is involved, the patient may develop delirium, paralysis and rapid death. Kidney damage is associated with the excretion of dark-colored urine (blackwater fever), hemoglobinuria, jaundice and acute renal failure. *P. vivax* infects only reticulocytes, and *P. malariae* infects only mature red blood cells. Persons whose genes carry the sickle cell trait are resistant to malaria because the ATPase of their red blood cells cannot produce sufficient energy for the growth of the malaria parasites. Also, most West Africans whose red blood cells lack the *P. vivex* Duffy blood group antigen Fy$^a$ or Fy$^b$ specific erythrocyte surface receptor are resistant to infection by *P. vivax*. An attack of malaria tends to produce a specific though partial immunity that seems to be due to the heightened activity of the fixed phagocytic cells.

## 3. Laboratory Diagnosis

Diagnosis of malaria is best made by microscopic examination of Giemsa-stained thin and thick peripheral blood smears. For example, in thin blood smears red blood cells parasitized with *P. malariae* are normal in size and they show parasitic band forms. The smears of red blood cells parasitized with *P. falciparum* show multiple rings and/or banana-shaped gametocytes. The thin smears of red blood cells parasitized with either *P. vivax* or *P. ovale* show red cells that typically oval, with Schuffner's dots and a ragged cell wall. Figure 6-1 shows red blood cells parasitized with *P. malariae, P. falciparum,* and *P. vivax.*

## 4. Treatment and Prevention

For sensitive strains of the malaria parasites, chloroquine is the drug of choice. However, dormant *P. vivax* and *P. ovale* in liver cells are not killed and require primaquine for their elimination. For malarial parasites that are resistant to the previous two drugs, mefloquine alone or in combination with quinine may be used. All of these antimalarial drugs interfere with DNA replication.

Prevention rests on the destruction of anopheles mosquitoes. This is best achieved by attacking the mosquito breeding areas with such measures as the use of insecticide sprays and draining and filling swamp ponds or other similar bodies of stagnant water. Adequate screening of houses is another reasonable way of reducing the incidence of malaria.

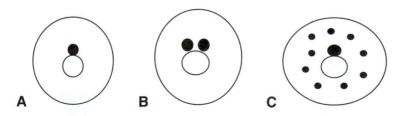

Figure 6-1. Red blood cells parasitized with (**A**) *P. malariae,* (**B**) *P. falciparum,* and (**C**) *P. vivax.*

### B. *Babesia microti* and *B. divergens*

These protozoa resemble the malaria parasites and cause babesiosis. This disease features irregular fever, chills, sweating, muscle pain, mild hepatosplenomegaly and possible hemolytic anemia. *Babesiosis* is transmitted to humans by tick bites. *Babesia* parasites enter red blood cells and may present a diagnostic problem for malaria.

Laboratory diagnosis rests on recognition of the parasite in infected red blood cells on peripheral blood. A Maltese cross within these cells is of diagnostic value.

Babesiosis can be treated with clindamycin and quinine.

## III. BLOOD AND TISSUE PROTOZOA

### A. *Trypanosoma cruzi, T. brucei rhodesiense, T. brucei gambiense*

#### 1. Transmission and Life Cycle

American trypanosomiasis or Chagas' disease, caused by *T. cruzi,* is transmitted to humans by reduviid bugs. African trypanosomiasis, caused by *T. b. rhodesiense* or *T. b. gambiense,* is transmitted to humans by blood-sucking tsetse flies of the genus *Glossina.* The body of trypanosomes suggests a diminutive dolphin (Fig. 6-2).

In the life cycle of *T. cruzi,* reduviid bugs (kissing bugs, or triatomids) take a blood meal from humans infected with *T. cruzi,* which exists either as a free, flagellated form called trypomastigote or as a nonflagellate form within macrophages known as amastigote. In the midgut of the reduviid bug, *T. cruzi* transforms to a flagellated stage, called the epimastigote, and then migrates to the hindgut, where it transforms into the infective trypomastigote form. These forms pass out of the reduviid bug in its feces, which is deposited during feeding, and can then be rubbed into the bite. The trypomastigotes are engulfed by macrophages and transform into amastigotes. The reservoirs of infection for *T. cruzi* include humans, raccoons, rats, armadillos, dogs and cats.

The life cycles of *T. b. rhodesiense* and *T. b. gambiense* involve the tsetse flies as vectors and humans and animals as reservoirs of infection. Trypomastigotes are ingested by tsetse flies, multiply in the midgut and then migrate to salivary glands, where further multiplication occurs as epimastigotes. Finally, epimastigotes transform into trypomastigotes prior to transmission to the vertebrate host.

#### 2. Pathogenesis and Clinical Manifestations

American trypanosomiasis begins with an edematous swelling of the eyelids and conjunctiva. The swelling is called chacoma. *T. cruzi* is then disseminated through the lymphatics and bloodstream to various muscles.

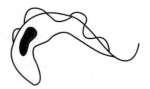

Figure 6-2.  Mature trypanosome.

The heart is most commonly affected. The heart changes include apical aneurisms, thinning of ventricular walls, mural thrombi, right bundle-branch block, tachycardia, bradycardia, cardiomyopathy or heart failure. Involvement of the gastrointestinal tract is associated with various degrees of dilation of the esophagus (megaesophagus) and colon (megacolon).

African trypanosomiasis begins with a self-limited inflammatory lesion about 1 week after the bite of a tsetse fly infected with either *T. b. rhodesiense* or *T. b. gambiense*. The trypanosomes then spread through the lymphatics and bloodstream, causing a febrile systemic illness with widespread lymphadenopathy and splenomegaly. The stage of the disease is known as stage I African trypanosomiasis. Stage II of African trypanosomiasis involves the central nervous system, and it is characterized by progressive indifference and daytime somnolence and thus it is called sleeping sickness. There is also speech impairment, ataxia and tremors resembling Parkinson's disease with progressive neurologic damage which can lead to coma and death. The pathogenesis of African trypanosomiasis is due to great antigenic variation of surface glycoproteins of trypanosomes which allow the organisms to evade the host immune response, because the lytic antibody formed by the host is directed against the surface glycoproteins.

### 3. Laboratory Diagnosis

The diagnosis of American trypanosomiasis may be made by microscopic examination of stained and wet preparations of fresh anticoagulated blood. If these efforts fail to demonstrate trypomastigotes, mouse inoculation, blood culture and xenodiagnosis may be successful. In xenodiagnosis uninfected reduviid bugs are allowed to feed on the patient's blood, and after about a month the intestinal material is examined for parasites.

In the early stages of African trypanosomiasis microscopic examination of stained and wet smears of stained and wet preparations of fresh blood or lymph aspirate may reveal trypomastigotes. The late stage of this disease may be diagnosed by the demonstration of trypanosomes in the spinal fluid and serological tests for the detection of IgM against *T. b. rhodesiense* or *T. b. gambiense*.

### 4. Treatment and Prevention

The only drug that is only partially effective against American trypanosomiasis is nifurtimox, which reduces the mortality rate, the duration of symptoms and the level of parasitemia. Stage I African trypanosomiasis responds to suramin, but once encephalitis of stage II sets in suramin is ineffective because it cannot pass the blood–brain barrier well. Prevention of Chagas' disease and sleeping sickness depends on the suppression of reduviid bugs and tsetse flies. The wearing of protective clothing, use of insect repellents and avoidance of areas that harbor infective trypanosomes may reduce the risk of Chagas' disease or sleeping sickness.

## B. *Leishmania donovani, L. tropica, L. mexicana, L. braziliensis*

### 1. Transmission and Life Cycle

In the circulating blood and cultures the leishmania organisms are flagellated but differ somewhat from the trypanosomes. In the infected body cells they lose their flagella and assume a typically rounded form. Transmission of leishmaniasis occurs by bites of the female sandflies of the genera Phlebotomus and Lutzomyia. The life cycle includes the sandfly feeding on an infected individual, whereby it takes up parasitized macrophages. Upon reaching the midgut of the sandfly, the nonflagellated amastigote form of the parasite transforms into the flagellated promastigote form of leishmania. After division, it reaches the buccal cavity of sandfly, from where it is injected into the skin of an individual. The promastigotes are taken up by the reticuloendothelial cells, where they transform into amastigotes and cycles again.

## 2. Pathogenesis and Clinical Manifestations

*L. donovani* is the cause of visceral leishmaniasis, or Kalb-azar. This organism attacks the fixed phagocytic cells of liver, spleen and bone marrow. This severe action of parasites on the reticuloendothelial system, especially in malnourished young children, causes fever, anorexia, weight loss, hepatomegaly, massive splenomegaly and abdominal distention with discomfort. Patients tend also to develop a severe anemia and a very low white cell count. Healing and resistance to *L. donovani, L. tropicana, L. mexicana* or *L. braziliensis* are associated with the Th cells, production of γ interferon and activation of macrophages to kill intracellular amastigotes. Liberation of lymphokines from sensitized T cells triggers host cell cytotoxicity and is believed to be the mechanism of pathogenesis of leishmania as well as trypanosomes.

*L. tropica* and *L. mexicana* both cause cutaneous leishmaniasis, while *L. braziliensis* is the etiological agent of mucocutaneous leishmaniasis.

Cutaneous leishmaniasis features a nodule formation at the site of bite of the sandfly which may either ulcerate or diffuse and form multiple nodules. Cutaneous leishmaniasis is confused with impetigo, sporotrichosis and mycobacterial infections. Mucocutaneous leishmaniasis starts with a skin ulcer, and then ulcers form at the mucous membranes of nose and mouth.

## 3. Laboratory Diagnosis

The diagnosis of leishmaniasis depends on the demonstration of the amastigotes in stained smears from skin lesions, blood, bone marrow and liver biopsies. A skin test is positive for cutaneous or mucocutaneous leishmaniasis but not for visceral leishmaniasis.

## 4. Treatment and Prevention

The drug of choice for the treatment of leishmaniasis is sodium stibogluconate, an antimonial compound that inactivates the sulfhydryl groups of proteins and enzymes.

Prevention depends on avoidance and control of sandflies by such means as use of protective clothing, use of insecticide spraying and screens or bed nets to keep out sandflies.

## C. *Toxoplasma gondii*

### 1. Transmission and Life Cycle

*T. gondii* is an intracellular, coccidial organism resembling the malaria parasites. The definitive host is the cat and other feline animals. Humans, mice, pigs and sheep serve as the intermediate host for the development of *T. gondii*. Human infection may occur by ingestion of raw sheep or pork meat containing oocysts of *T. gondii,* by inhalation of oocysts from cat feces or congenitally if a pregnant woman is exposed to toxoplasma for the first time. Certain toxoplasma forms called trophozoites produced by oocysts have a crescentic, slender shape and are called tachyzoites. They multiply rapidly and are responsible for the initial infection and tissue damage. Short, slowly growing trophozoites are called bradyzoites and are involved in chronic toxoplasmosis.

## 2. Pathogenesis and Clinical Manifestations

The main organs affected by tachyzoites are the lymphatic tissue, myocardium, the central nervous system, retina, placenta and skeletal muscle, where the toxoplasma causes an acute inflammatory response, cell death and focal necrosis. The parasites also cause an increased level of IgA, activation of macrophages, γ interferon production and stimulation of cytotoxic CD8 T lymphocytes. Patients infected with the human immunodeficiency virus, who have had an organ transplant or who have taken immunosuppressive drugs are most likely to develop disseminated, or central nervous system, toxoplasmosis. In healthy persons most infections are benign or asymptomatic. When acute illness occurs it consists of chills, fever, headache, myalgia, lymphadenitis and fatigue. Chronic disease may feature, lymphadenitis, rash, encephalomyelitis, hepatitis or chorioretinitis. Congenital infection may cause epilepsy, spontaneous abortion, stillbirth, blindness, mental retardation, encephalitis, microcephaly or hydrocephalus.

## 3. Laboratory Diagnosis

The diagnosis of toxoplasmosis depends on the inoculation of blood or other body fluids into mice and the isolation of toxoplasma parasites from the peritoneal cavity 1–2 weeks after inoculation. Other diagnostic tests include demonstration of high antibody titers against toxoplasma and radiological tests such as CT and MRI for the demonstration of focal and multifocal abnormalities in patients with toxoplasmic encephalitis.

## 4. Treatment and Prevention

Toxoplasmosis can be treated with pyrimethamine plus either sulfadiazine or clindamycin. Pyrimethamine and sulfadiazine in combination block folic acid synthesis and thus reduce the parasitic host population.

Prevention depends on proper cooking of meat and by avoiding oocyst contaminated material, i.e., the cat's litter box.

# IV. INTESTINAL AND UROGENITAL PROTOZOA

## A. *Entamoeba histolytica*

### 1. Transmission and Life Cycle

*E. histolytica* exists as a trophozoite and a cyst, and humans are the main hosts and reservoirs of *E. histolytica.* The trophozoites vary in diameter from 10 to 30 μ, move very rapidly in a straight line and contain ingested red blood cells; their nucleus is very delicate, and its nuclear membrane is encrusted with uniform fine chromatin granules. When preparing to encyst, the amebas become smaller, rounded and lay down a delicate cyst wall. The large nucleus then divides progressively into four small nuclei. Figure 6-3 shows a trophozoite and a cyst of *E. histolytica*.

Amebiasis is usually transmitted by direct person-to-person fecal–oral spread under conditions of poor personal hygiene. Food and water spread may result in epidemic amebiasis. Venereal transmission is also known to occur in male homosexuals as a result of oral–anal sexual contact.

The life cycle of *E. histolytica* begins with the ingestion of cysts, as trophozoites die quickly outside the intestinal tract. After ingestion of cysts and passage through the stomach, the cysts reach the distal small bowel, the cyst cell wall lyses and the parasites that are released transform to trophozoites and are carried to colon. The trophozoites multiply asexually by binary fission and change to resistant, infective cysts, which are passed in feces (trophozoites may be found in fresh, fluid or soft feces).

## 2. Pathogenesis and Clinical Manifestations

In harmony with parasitic infections, amebiasis is prevalent in tropical Asia, Africa and Central and South America. In the United States, 1–5% of the population harbors *E. histolytica*. However, the majority of these individuals are colonized with strains of amebas that are of low virulence and that remain in the intestine as harmless commensals. Occasionally they may invade tissue and cause tissue damage. Synthesis of an extracellular cysteine proteinase, which digests secretory IgA, elastin and collagen, and of phospholipase A and a host cell membrane pore-forming peptides has been associated with the conversion of an avirulent strain of *E. histolytica* to a virulent one. Immunity is incomplete and does not correlate with antibody response. Amebas lyse colonic epithelial cells and produce mucosal ulcerations, which when extensive can lead to secondary bacterial infection. *E. histolytica* may also enter the portal circulation and when carried to the liver, lung, brain or spleen, cause rarely liquefaction necrosis and formation of abscess cavities. The most common symptoms are abdominal pain, nausea, flatulence and bowel irregularity with headaches, fatigue and nervousness in a minority of cases. These symptoms can be confused with many other gastrointestinal disorders. The diarrhea is intermittent over months to years. The stools are watery, foul-smelling and contain mucus and blood. Fulminating amebic dysentery is less common and features high fever, severe abdominal cramps and profuse, bloody diarrhea with tenesmus.

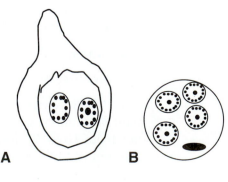

Figure 6-3. *Entamoeba histolytica:*
(**A**) Trophozoite and (**B**) cyst.    **A**          **B**

### 3. Laboratory Diagnosis

Definitive diagnosis of intestinal amebiasis requires the demonstration of blood containing motile trophozoites or small, round cysts with four nuclei in fresh stools. An indirect hemagglutination test is routinely positive for invasive amebiasis. Finally, an enzyme immunoassay can detect *E. histolytica* antigen in stool.

### 4. Treatment and Prevention

The drug of choice for the treatment of intestinal or liver abscesses is metronidazole combined with iodoquinol.

Prevention of amebiasis rests on sanitation and protection of water and food, especially vegetables, from pollution. Careful washing of hands with soap and water after using the toilet can also reduce the incidence of amebiasis. This hand washing applies particularly to food handlers and to institutionalized patients.

## B. *Giardia lamblia*

### 1. Transmission and Life Cycle

*G. lamblia* can be found in the human, animal, bird or amphibian intestine as a trophozoite and a cyst. The trophozoite resembles a tennis racket without a handle. Figure 6-4 illustrates the fantastic morphology of *G. lamblia*. Giardiasis is acquired by the ingestion of the cyst in contaminated food or water. Once the cyst is ingested, it undergoes exocystation in the small intestine and forms two trophozoites.

### 2. Pathogenesis and Clinical Manifestations

Following ingestion of cysts and conversion to trophozoites, *G. lamblia* attaches to the duodenum, where it may cause inflammation and malabsorption of fat and protein. The patients develop a nonbloody, foul-smelling, greasy, frothy diarrhea along with abdominal gassy distention and cramps. Many patients become asymptomatic chronic carriers and excrete cysts for years.

### 3. Laboratory Diagnosis

The diagnosis of giardiasis rests on the demonstration of typical trophozoites or cysts in the stools.

### 4. Treatment and Prevention

The drug of choice is metronidazole. Prevention depends on consumption of uncontaminated food or water and proper cooking as well as handling of food.

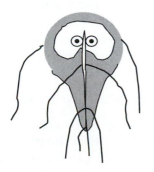

Figure 6-4. *Giardia lamblia* trophozoite.

## C. *Cryptosporidium parvum* and *Isospora belli*

### 1. Transmission and Life Cycle

These organisms are the smallest (2–6 μm), oval or spherical, obligate intracellular parasites that live in human and animal intestinal cells. The infective oocysts are excreted in the stool of parasitized hosts. After ingestion by an individual or animal, sporozoites are released and attach to the bowel epithelial cells, where they are changed to trophozoites. These divide asexually to form schizonts, each of which first contains type I merozoites and eventually type II merozoites. Type II merozoites, upon release from schizonts, form male and female gametocytes. Following fertilization, the resulting zygote develops into an oocyst, and it is shed in the lumen of the bowel and then excreted in stools. Transmission occurs by ingestion of the oocysts.

### 2. Pathogenesis and Clinical Manifestations

Both *Cryptosporidium parvum* and *Isospora belli* can cause diarrhea in both immunocompetent and immunocompromised patients. The majority of infections are asymptomatic in individuals with intact immune systems as well as in persons with immunological deficiencies. However, cryptosporidiosis and isosporiasis tend to be particularly common and chronic in AIDS patients, while these infections are infrequent and acute in immunocompetent individuals. The clinical manifestations of cryptosporidiasis and isosporiasis are similar and include watery, nonbloody diarrhea, anorexia, weight loss, fever and possible abdominal pain.

### 3. Laboratory Diagnosis

The diagnosis of cryptosporidiasis and isosporiasis rests on the demonstration of vary small (4–6 μm), acid-fast oocysts in stools and direct immunofluorescent stains for *C. parvum* or *I. belli* oocysts.

### 4. Treatment and Prevention

Chemotherapeutic drugs are ineffective against cryptosporidiasis, but isosporiasis responds to trimethoprim-sulfamethoxazole. Supportive treatment includes administration of antidiarrheal drugs plus fluid and electrolyte replacement.

Prevention rests on proper water filtration for the removal of oocysts, which are resistant to water chlorination.

## D. *Naegleria fowleri* and *Acanthamoeba castellani*

### 1. Transmission and Life Cycle

*N. fowleri* and *A. castellani* exist as free-living trophozoites and cysts. They live in soil or fresh water. Transmission to humans occurs by aspiration of water containing trophozoites or cysts and by inhalation of contaminated dust. Following invasion of the olfactory neuroepithelium, they migrate to the brain and cause meningoencephalitis.

### 2. Pathogenesis and Clinical Manifestations

*N. fowleri* produces purulent meningitis and encephalitis, while *A. castellani* is also associated with keratitis. Primary amoebic meningoencephalitis features high fever, severe headache, nausea, vomiting, photophobia, seizures and coma, and death may follow. Keratitis results from microscopic eye damage from contaminated contact lenses. Surface eye infection causes corneal abscesses, while deep infection and lead to loss of vision.

### 3. Laboratory Diagnosis

Diagnosis rests on the detection of *N. fowleri*, or *A. castellani* trophozoites in fresh, wet mounts of spinal fluid or of corneal abscess clinical specimens.

### 4. Treatment and Prevention

In few instances, treatment with amphotericin B has been successful. For keratitis, a combination of chemotherapy and corneal transplantation may be effective. Prevention is very problematic, but filtration of swimming pool water and proper use and disinfection of contact lenses may reduce the incidence of keratitis.

## E. *Trichomonas vaginalis*

### 1. Transmission and Life Cycle

*T. vaginalis* is a pear-shaped protozoan 5–30 µm long and 2–14 µm wide. This organism has four anterior flagella, an undulating membrane, an elongated nucleus and a rod (axostyle) that starts at the base of flagella and protrudes through the posterior end of *T. vaginalis*. This parasite does not produce a cyst but can survive few hours outside its human host. Trichomoniasis is usually transmitted by sexual intercourse. Transmission of organisms by contaminated shared washcloths or infection of neonates by passage through an infected birth canal is uncommon. The prevalence of trichomoniasis is linked to sexual activity. It is estimated that 5–7 million women in the United States acquire this disease annually, and 30–70% of their sexual male partners may also be infected. The life cycle of *T. vaginalis* involves its migration to the vagina and prostate following sexual intercourse.

### 2. Pathogenesis and Clinical Manifestations

Changes in the pH of vagina, hormonal levels and alterations in the physiology of *T. vaginalis* may be involved in the modulation of the severity of pathologic changes of vagina, prostate or other organs of the human genitourinary tract. Humoral, secretory and cellular immune reactions are present in patients with trichomoniasis, but there is no significant immunity to trichomoniasis. The majority of men infected with *T. vaginalis* remain asymptomatic, and few develop prostatitis or epididymitis. Women infected with this protozoan usually are symptomatic. Thus, they have a foul-smelling, yellow-green, profuse, frothy vaginal discharge, vulvar erythema and itching, dysuria or urinary frequency.

### 3. Laboratory Diagnosis

Diagnosis depends on the microscopic demonstration of *T. vaginalis* motile *trophozoites* in wet mounts of vaginal or prostatic specimens, direct immunofluorescent staining for *T. vaginalis* and culture of this organism.

### 4. Treatment and Prevention

Metronidazole for treatment; use of condoms for prevention.

## V. INTESTINAL NEMATHELMINTHES (ROUNDWORMS)

### A. *Enterobius vermicularis* (Pinworm)

#### 1. Transmission and Life Cycle

*E. vermicularis* is a 10-mm spindle-shaped, roundworm with a tough outer cuticle and a sharply pointed tail resembling a pin. The female worm produces eggs that are clear, thin-walled, flattened on one side and usually embryonated (Fig. 6-5).

Transmission of enterobiasis occurs most frequently by the ingestion of eggs. *E. vermicularis* has a simple fecal–oral cycle with no extra intestinal migration, and it is confined to humans. After the pinworm eggs are ingested by an individual they hatch, and larvae mature to adults in the intestine. The adults mate in the cecum, and the female worm migrates at night to the perineal area where it deposits many thousands of eggs that are excreted in the environment during defecation. This cycle is then repeated.

#### 2. Pathogenesis and Clinical Manifestations

Enterobiasis is widespread. In the United States millions of persons have been estimated to be infected with *E. vermicularis*. However, the adult pinworms fail to produce significant pathologic changes in the intestine, and they also appear to be incapable of inducing protective immunity. The principal clinical manifestation is perineal itching.

#### 3. Laboratory Diagnosis

The diagnosis rests on the demonstration of eggs of *E. vermicularis* from the anal mucosa with a low-power microscope. Worms, not eggs, are found in stools.

#### 4. Treatment and Prevention

Patients with enterobiasis as well as their cohabitants should be treated with pyrantel pamoate and mebendazole for several weeks. Pyrantel pamoate inhibits fumarate reductase and blocks neuromuscular action, which leads to pinworm paralysis. Mebendazole, and the related drugs thiabendazole and albendazole, inhibits fumarase reductase and glucose transport and disrupts microtubular function. There are no effective preventive measures.

### B. *Trichuris trichuria* (Whipworm)

#### 1. Transmission and Life Cycle

*T. trichuria* is an approximately 40-mm long roundworm. Its anterior two-thirds is thin, while its rear end is thick, resembling a minute whip from which it derives its name (whipworm). The female worm produces

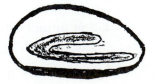

Figure 6-5. Embryonated egg of *Enterobius vermicularis*.

thousands of eggs daily. The eggs are brown and have opercular, translucent plugs at both ends (Fig. 6-6).

Whipworms are common inhabitants of the cecum and large intestine of humans and animals. They are usually transmitted by ingestion of ova of *T. trichuria*. The life cycle of the whipworm is similar to that of *E. vermicularis*, the main difference being that the eggs of *T. trichuria* are passed in the stools and have to be incubated in the soil before they become infective.

### 2. Pathogenesis and Clinical Manifestations

The adult whipworms attach to the intestinal mucosa and may cause ulceration and hemorrhage. The ulcers allow enteric bacteria to enter the blood stream and cause bacteremia. IgE antibodies develop following infection, but they cannot induce significant immunity to *T. trichuria*. Most infections are asymptomatic. When the whipworm load is sufficient the patients experience abdominal pain, diarrhea, nausea, stunting of growth and anemia. A modest eosinophilia is also common in these infections.

### 3. Laboratory Diagnosis

Diagnosis rests on the microscopic demonstration of brown, lemon-shaped eggs of *T. trichuris* that have plugs at both ends.

### 4. Treatment and Prevention

The drug of choice is mebendazole. Prevention depends on proper disposal of fecal material and good personal hygiene.

## C. *Ascaris lumbricoides*

### 1. Transmission and Life Cycle

*A. lumbricoides* is the largest of the usual intestinal worms, measuring 150–350 mm. Its firm, creamy cuticle and pointed anterior and posterior ends differentiate it from the common earthworm. The eggs are elliptic in shape and have a thick, clear inner shell covered with a warty albuminous coat. Transmission of ascariasis occurs usually by ingestion of egg-contaminated food or soil and by inhalation of dust containing eggs of *A. lumbricoides*. The life cycle of this roundworm is similar to *T. trichuria*, the only key difference being that, after hatching from the egg in the intestinal lumen, ascarid larvae penetrate the bowel wall and then move to the liver and lung before returning to the intestinal lumen.

### 2. Pathogenesis and Clinical Manifestations

The severity of pulmonary damage induced by the migration of larvae through the lungs appears to be related in part to an immediate hypersensitivity reaction to larval antigens. Pulmonary infection may be asso-

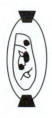

Figure 6-6.  Egg of *Trichuris trichuria*.

ciated with such clinical manifestations as irritating nonproductive cough, burning substernal discomfort, fever, eosinophilia, apnea, and blood-tinged sputum. Heavy intestinal infections may be associated with rectal pain, small bowel obstruction or perforation, intussusception and volvulus. Also, a single large worm can enter and block the biliary tree, causing colic, cholecystitis, cholangitis, pancreatitis and hepatic abscesses.

### 3. Laboratory Diagnosis

The vast majority of cases of ascariasis can be diagnosed by microscopic demonstration of the characteristic warty eggs of *A. lumbricoides* in fecal clinical samples.

### 4. Treatment and Prevention

The drug of choice for the treatment of ascariasis is mebendazole or albendazole. Intestinal or other organ obstructions require surgical intervention. Prevention of ascariasis requires proper disposal of fecal material and solid personal hygiene.

## D. *Necator americanus* and *Ancylostoma duodenale* (Hookworms)

### 1. Transmission and Life Cycle

These species of hookworms are identical, and both infect humans. *N. americanus* is found in Asia, Africa and America; *A. duodenale* is found in the Mediterranean basin, Middle East, India, China and Japan. The hookworms are pink-white and 10 mm long. The oral cavity of the hookworm contains sharp tooth-like structures, or cutting plates. The ova of *N. americanus* and *A. duodenale* have a thin shell and they are in a divisional stage as shown in Figure 6-7.

Transmission of hookworm disease occurs by skin penetration of filariform larvae that are part of the life cycle of *N. americanus* and *A. duodenale*. The life cycle of these hookworms begins with the production of eggs in the intestine. The eggs are then excreted with feces in soil, where rhabditiform larvae hatch and develop within a week into infective filariform larvae. Upon contact with human skin, filariform larvae penetrate the epidermis and reach the lungs by way of the blood stream. Here they rupture into alveolar spaces, are coughed up and swallowed and move into the small intestine, where they become adult hookworms.

### 2. Pathogenesis and Clinical Manifestations

The main pathological damage is loss of blood. The vast majority of hookworm infection is asymptomatic. Itchy maculopapular dermatitis may occur at the site where filariform larvae penetrate the skin. In some

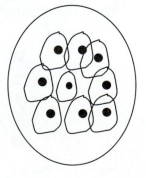

Figure 6-7. Hookworm egg, shown in a divisional stage.

instances larvae may cause pneumonitis when they migrate through the lungs. Other possible clinical manifestations include eosinophilia, inflammatory diarrhea, shortness of breath, hypoproteinemia, skin depigmentation and epigastric pain. The key feature of chronic hookworm disease is iron deficiency.

### 3. Laboratory Diagnosis

The diagnosis depends on the demonstration of hookworm eggs in human feces.

### 4. Treatment and Prevention

The drugs of choice are pyrantel pamoate and mebendazole. Management of anemia may require iron replacement or blood transfusion.

Prevention depends on improved sanitation.

## E. *Strongyloides stercoralis*

### 1. Transmission and Life Cycle

*S. stercoralis* is the smallest (2 mm) intestinal nematode. Its eggs are smaller but are similar to hookworm ova. Strongyloidiasis is the result of human skin penetration by the infective filariform larvae of *S. stercoralis* or of autoinfection. Thus, this roundworm has two life cycles. That is, the free-living cycle, which is similar to that found in hookworms, and the autoinfection cycle. In the second cycle, the exit of rhabditiform larvae to the environment is suppressed by constipation or other factors, and rhabditiform larvae transform to infective filariform larvae while they are still in the human body. The filariform larvae will then migrate through the lung back to the upper small bowel (autoinfection).

### 2. Pathogenesis and Clinical Manifestations

Damage to intestinal mucosa may cause inflammation, ulceration, malabsorption and abscess formation and may alter intestinal motility. Immunosuppression enhances risk of autoinfection by accelerating larval formation. Strongyloidiasis does not appear to induce any meaningful protective immunity. The clinical symptoms resemble those observed in hookworm infection, and eosinophilia is very common.

### 3. Laboratory Diagnosis

Diagnosis depends on the demonstration of rhabditiform larvae in fresh stools, in duodenal aspirates or in jejunal biopsy specimens.

### 4. Treatment and Prevention

The drug of choice for the treatment of strongyloidiasis is thiabendazole. Prevention of this disease depends on proper sewage disposal, use of shoes, gloves or other protective clothing and following good personal hygiene.

## F. *Trichinella spiralis*

### 1. Transmission and Life Cycle

*T. spiralis* is a whitish, 2–4 mm long, spirally shaped nematode that exists as a larva or a lemon-shaped cyst. Figure 6-8 shows larvae enclosed in a cyst.

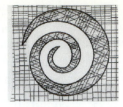

Figure 6-8.  *Trichinella spiralis* encysted
in pork striated muscle fibers.

Individuals usually acquire trichinosis by eating raw or improperly
cooked infected pork meat. Swine become infected by ingesting rats or
contaminated meat in garbage. The life cycle of *T. spiralis* features the
consumption of encysted larvae in pork and the excystment and maturation of larvae to adult worms in the intestinal mucosa, with the subsequent mating and production of eggs. The ova then hatch, and larvae
are released and spread by the bloodstream throughout the body. Only
larvae penetrating striated muscle survive. These larvae encyst and can
be excreted in stools, or they can remain encysted in striated muscle for
few years and then finally calcify.

### 2. Pathogenesis and Clinical Manifestations

The main pathological changes that occur in trichinosis are enlarge-
ment and/or loss of cross striations and basophilic degeneration of
muscle cells. The key symptoms of trichinosis include eosinophilia, periorbital edema, fever, muscular pains and diarrhea.

### 3. Laboratory Diagnosis

The diagnosis of trichinosis rests on the demonstration of larvae in
striated muscle by tissue biopsy. Also, the bentonite flocculation test for
*T. spiralis* is positive after the third week of illness.

### 4. Treatment and Prevention

Mebendazole or thiobendazole is effective against young larvae. Prevention depends on proper cooking of pork.

## VI. TISSUE FILARIAL NEMATHELMINTHES: *WUCHERERIA BANCROFTI, ONCHOCERCA VOLVULUS, LOA LOA*

### A. *Wuchereria bancrofti*

#### 1. Transmission and Life Cycle

*W. bancrofti* is a sheathed filarial worm 225–300 μm by 10 μm; it stains
red with Giemsa stain; its tail end tapers evenly, and it lacks nuclei. It is
transmitted to humans by bites of certain species of the female *Culex,
Anopheles* or *Aedes* mosquitoes. The definitive host for *W. bancrofti* is an
individual, wherein the adult worms live in the lymphatic channels or
lymph nodes. There the adult worm gives birth to microfilariae. Further
development of microfilariae requires the ingestion of these young larvae by a *Culex, Anopheles* or *Aedes* mosquito that serves as the intermediate
host. After the microfilariae are ingested by a mosquito, they penetrate
the stomach and migrate to breast muscle, where they transform into

infective larvae. The infective larvae then move into the proboscis of the mosquito and are introduced into the human skin by the mosquito bites.

### 2. Pathogenesis and Clinical Manifestations

The main pathological condition induced by filariasis is lymphatic obstruction, and it is due to numerous adult filarial worms as well as the immune responses. Infection requires extended exposure to *W. bancrofti,* which as a result causes chronic disease. The majority of infected individuals show light asymptomatic infection. Other patients have lymphangitis and lymphadenitis which subsides and recurs. They may also have headache, back pain and little fever associated with circulating microfilariae. Chronic disease leads to elephantiasis of legs, genitalia, breast and intra-abdominal lymphatics.

### 3. Laboratory Diagnosis

Diagnosis depends on the demonstration of microfilariae in blood smears. Blood specimens must be taken during the night because *W. bancrofti* circulates in the blood only at night.

### 4. Treatment and Prevention

Elimination of microfilariae from blood can be achieved with diethylcarbamazine, which causes neuromuscular paralysis. However, this drug has limited action on adult worms. Lymphatic obstruction requires surgical intervention. Prevention rests on effective mosquito control.

## B. *Onchocerca volvulus*

### 1. Transmission and Life Cycle

*O. volvulus* is a very long, filarial worm 20–700 mm by 0.2–0.4 mm. The microfilariae are sharp-tailed and unsheathed. *O. volvulus* differs from other human microfilariae in that they localize in the skin and eyes. *O. vulvulus* is usually enclosed in tough fibrous cysts or nodules. Human infection occurs by injection of infective larvae into the skin by black flies of the genus *Simulium.* The larvae migrate to subcutaneous tissues and develop to adult worms. The male and female worms become enclosed in subcutaneous nodules. Following fertilization, the female worms produces unsheathed microfilariae, which migrate to the skin, eyes and other tissues. Black flies that feed on humans can become infected and then transmit onchocerciasis.

### 2. Pathogenesis and Clinical Manifestations

The proteins of *O. vulvulus* cause acute and chronic inflammatory reactions in human tissues where they reside, giving rise to nodule formation, loss of subcutaneous elastic fibers and vision impairment. Patients with onchocerciasis may experience fever, eosinophilia, urticaria, wrinkling, thickening and pigmentation of skin, sclerosing keratitis, uveitis, chorioretinitis and optic neuritis.

### 3. Laboratory Diagnosis

Onchocerciasis can be diagnosed by the demonstration of adult worms of *O. vulvulus* in an excised nodule or of microfilariae in a skin biopsy specimen.

## 4. Treatment and Prevention

Invertin is effective against microfilariae. It blocks neuromuscular action. Suramin, which inhibits glycerol phosphate oxidase, can be curative, but it must be closely monitored for nephrotoxicity. Nodules on the head should be removed by surgical excision. Prevention rests on the control of black flies by insecticides and use of protective clothes.

## C. *Loa loa* (Eyeworm)

### 1. Transmission and Life Cycle

*L. loa* is a filarial worm with a sheath that does not stain with Giemsa. It has a short, recurved tail with nuclei in its tip. The adult worms and their microfilariae are as long as those of *W. bancrofti* (20–30 mm and 225–300 µm, respectively). Adult worms live in subcutaneous tissues, while microfilariae circulate in blood. Individuals acquire loiasis from infected biting flies of the genus *Chrysops,* which serve as the intermediate hosts. The microfilariae develop in the fly's abdomen, become infective and invade the proboscis, which introduces infective microfilariae into human skin.

### 2. Pathogenesis and Clinical Manifestations

The creeping, painless, itchy swellings in the skin known as Calabar swellings that are caused by the migration are believed to be induced by allergic reactions to *L. loa* proteins and its metabolic products. Loiasis is often clinically recognized by the presence of Calabar swellings, painful congestion, inflammation of conjunctiva, edema of eyelids and impaired vision.

### 3. Laboratory Diagnosis

Loiasis can be diagnosed by the demonstration of microfilariae in the peripheral blood or by the isolation of adult eye worm from the eye.

### 4. Treatment and Prevention

Repeated administration of diethylcarbamazine is recommended for the treatment of loiasis. Prevention rests on the control of biting flies and use of protective clothing.

## D. *Dracunculus medinensis* (Guinea worm)

### 1. Transmission and Life Cycle

*D. medinensis* is transmitted to humans by ingestion of the minute freshwater crustaceans infected with larvae of the Guinea worm. The larvae penetrate the intestinal wall and move to subcutaneous tissues, where the larvae mature into adults and mate. Within a year the female worm can grow to 100 cm; it migrates to human skin, and a portion of its body, which includes its uterus, exits the skin. When its uterus comes in contact with water, it releases motile larvae, which infect the crustaceans.

### 2. Pathogenesis and Clinical Manifestations

The pathological features and clinical symptoms of dracunculosis are limited to possible allergic reactions including urticaria, fever, periorbital edema, local pain and swelling.

### 3. Laboratory Diagnosis

Dracunculosis can be diagnosed by the demonstration of *D. medinensis* in human tissues.

### 4. Treatment and Prevention

Gradual removal, or surgical excision of the Guinea worm. Dracunculosis may be prevented by the availability of safe drinking water.

## E. *Toxocara canis*

### 1. Transmission and Life Cycle

*T. canis* exists as an infective egg, larva and an adult dog nematode. Humans acquire toxocariasis, or visceral larva migrans, by ingestion of *T. canis* ova from canine stools. The life cycle of the dog worm is very similar to that of *Ascaris lumbricoides*.

### 2. Pathogenesis and Clinical Manifestations

Larvae of *T. canis* induce necrosis, bleeding and formation of eosinophilic granulomas. The organs commonly involved are the lungs, heart, liver, eye, skeletal muscle and brain. However, the majority of infections in humans and canine animals are asymptomatic.

### 3. Laboratory Diagnosis

The diagnosis of toxocariasis is made by the demonstration of the dog worm larvae in liver biopsy specimens.

### 4. Treatment and Prevention

Administration of diethylcarbamazine, and corticosteroids for serious pulmonary, myocardial and nervous system involvement. Prevention depends on deworming of dogs.

## VII. PLATYHELMINTHES (FLATWORMS)—CESTODES

### A. *Taenia saginata* (Beef Tapeworm)

#### 1. Transmission and Cycle

Cestodes are long, ribbon-like worms that lack vascular, respiratory and intestinal systems. Their body consists of a head or scolex equipped with muscular suckers used for attachment to intestinal mucosa of its host. Some species have an additional attachment head structure with hooks, referred to as the rostellum. Behind the scolex is a neck, from which body segments known as proglottids are formed. Every proglottid is a complete hermaphroditic reproductive unit which is connected to other hundreds or thousands proglottids by a common cuticle, excretory canals and nerves. When a proglottid becomes gravid, it releases its eggs (see Fig. 6-9).

Humans are the only definitive hosts for the adult beef tapeworm which lives in the intestinal tract. Cattle is the common intermediate host. The life cycle of *T. saginata* includes three basic morphological forms: adult → ovum → larva (cysticercus). The adult tapeworm produces eggs in the human intestinal tract, and these eggs are deposited on vegetation.

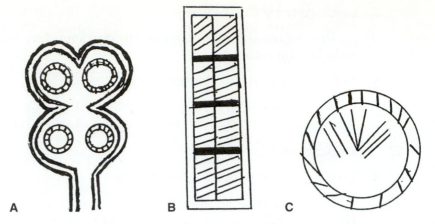

Figure 6-9. *Taenia saginata:* (**A**) scolex; (**B**) proglottid; (**C**) ovum.

Cattle feeding on the vegetation allow the ova to enter the bovine intestinal tract, move to striated muscle and transform to cysticerci. Human transmission of *T. saginata* occurs by ingestion of improperly cooked beef containing cysticerci, which later become adult tapeworms.

### 2. Pathogenesis and Clinical Manifestations

The pathological and clinical symptoms of taeniasis include presence of the adult beef tapeworm in the human intestinal tract with such minor clinical signs as mild abdominal pain or discomfort. Elevated levels of IgE and eosinophilia may also be present.

### 3. Laboratory Diagnosis

Taeniasis due to *T. saginata* can be diagnosed by the detection of proglottids, ova or scolex of beef tapeworm in fecal or cellophane-tape human specimens.

### 4. Treatment and Prevention

Praziquantel is very effective for therapy. Prevention depends upon proper cooking of beef, beef inspection and suitable disposal of human feces.

## B. *Taenia solium (Pork Tapeworm)*

### 1. Transmission and Life Cycle

The morphology of *T. solium* is closely similar to that of *T. saginata* except that the proglottids of the pork tapeworm are less elongated than those of the beef tapeworm. Also, *T. solium* has two rows of hookers on its rostellum. Transmission of the pork tapeworm occurs by ingestion of undercooked pork infected with cysticerci of *T. solium*. The life cycle of the pork tapeworm resembles that of *T. saginata,* except that human cysticercosis may result from ingestion of eggs of *T. solium* either from fecally contaminated food or by autoinfection. Thus humans can serve both as definitive and intermediate hosts for adult worms or larvae (cysticerci).

### 2. Pathogenesis and Clinical Manifestations

Pork tapeworm intestinal infections may be asymptomatic or may include such symptoms as abdominal discomfort, nausea, diarrhea or weight loss. Cysticercosis patients can have any organ infected with cysticerci, but the brain is usually involved. Thus, clinical manifestations may include headache, dizziness, ataxia, vomiting, visual changes, confusion, hydrocephalus, meningitis and seizures.

### 3. Laboratory Diagnosis

Adult worm intestinal infections are diagnosed as described for *T. saginata*. The diagnosis of cysticercosis is confirmed by demonstration of cysticerci in a clinical biopsy specimen. Computed tomography (CT) and magnetic resonance imaging (MRI) may identify active or calcified lesions of cysticercosis.

### 4. Treatment and Prevention

Intestinal infection caused by *T. solium* is treated with praziquantel. The management of neurocysticercosis requires combined therapy with praziquantel and albendazole. It may also require surgery and use of glucocorticosteroids. Prevention of *T. solium* rests upon adequate cooking of pork, suitable inspection of pork products and proper treatment of human feces.

## C. *Diphyllobothrium latum* (Fish Tapeworm)

### 1. Transmission and Life Cycle

*D. latum* has an elongated scolex, and in contrast to other cestodes its scolex features sucking grooves instead of suckers. The ova of the fish tapeworm are oval and have an operculum (lid). Transmission of *D. latum* occurs by ingestion of raw or improperly cooked fish infected with larvae of this tapeworm. The life cycle of the fish tapeworm involves the release of ova into water and their hatching and consumption by freshwater crustaceans. After an infected crustacean is ingested by a fish, the young larvae (procercoids) migrate to fish muscle and develop to mature larvae (plerocercoids, or sparganum larvae). These plerocercoids are swallowed by humans and develop into adult worms, which produce numerous eggs.

### 2. Pathogenesis and Clinical Manifestations

The main pathological finding is the presence of fish tapeworms in the human intestine with some inflammation. Most of *D. latum* infections are asymptomatic, but they may be associated with occasional abdominal discomfort, weight loss, weakness and diarrhea. In very few instances the fish tapeworm can cause megaloblastic anemia in the elderly because *D. latum* may absorb large amounts of vitamin $B_{12}$.

### 3. Laboratory Diagnosis

Definitive diagnosis requires the demonstration of operculated ova in stool or proglottids that are wider than long in feces or vomitus.

### 4. Treatment and Prevention

Diphyllobothriasis may be managed with praziquantel. Megaloblastic anemia can be treated with administration of vitamin $B_{12}$. Prevention depends upon proper cooking of fish and suitable human fecal sanitation.

### D. *Echinococcus granulosus* (Dog Tapeworm)

#### 1. Transmission and Life Cycle

*E. granulosus* is the smallest cestode (5 mm), and it contains only three proglottids. The dog tapeworm forms hydatid cysts around its larvae. These cysts are filled with fluid and are composed of an external laminated cuticle and an internal germinal membrane. Daughter cysts form inside the original ones, and within each of these daughter cysts new protoscolices are generated from the germinal membrane. Few settle to the bottom of the cyst and form what is known as hydatid sand. Transmission of echinococcosis occurs by the ingestion of eggs of *E. granulosus*. The main events in the life cycle of *E. granulosus* include the residence of adult worms in the intestine of dogs or other canine animals, production of eggs and their excretion in dog stool. After ingestion of eggs by an intermediate host such as an individual, sheep, cattle, horse, pig or elk, larvae emerge. These migrate and concentrate in the liver, lung and brain and form hydatid cysts.

#### 2. Pathogenesis and Clinical Manifestations

Echinococcal hydatid cysts that are small, or grow slowly, do not cause any tissue damage or symptoms. However, within 5–20 years they can enlarge and induce clinical manifestations either by organ compression or by breakage of cysts and release of hydatid fluid that induces immediate allergic reactions. Thus, patients with echinococcosis present with abdominal pain, a palpable mass in the upper right quadrant, biliary obstruction, jaundice, fever, itching, anaphylaxis, urticaria and eosinophilia.

Related echinococci such as *E. multilocaris* or *E. vogeli* can also cause echinococcosis.

#### 3. Laboratory Diagnosis

Computed tomography guided aspiration of hydatid cyst fluid and demonstration of scoliceal hookers. Detection of *E. granulosus* DNA in biopsy specimens by DNA probes. MRI, CT and ultrasound tests may reveal well-defined cysts.

#### 4. Treatment and Prevention

If possible, excision of cysts is the definitive treatment. However, extreme caution must be taken to avoid possible anaphylaxis from leakage of hydatid cyst fluid. Treatment with high doses of albendazole, bemendazole or praziquantel may be considered when the location of hydatid cyst does not permit surgical intervention. Prevention depends upon such measures as not allowing dogs in the vicinity of animal slaughter, not permitting them to feed on viscera of slain sheep or other animals and elimination of stray dogs.

### E. *Hymenolepis nana* (Dwarf Tapeworm)

#### 1. Transmission and Life Cycle

*H. nana* is a dwarf (1.5–5.0 cm) cestode, and it produces characteristic eggs with six-hooked embryos and polar filaments. This flatworm is transmitted to humans by ingestion of embryonated eggs or by autoinfection. *H. nana* has a simple life cycle and does not require an intermediate host. The ingested eggs transform to cysticercoid larvae in the intestinal villi, and then these larvae become adult worms, which produce infective ova that are excreted in feces.

### 2. Pathogenesis and Clinical Manifestations

The only pathological manifestation is the presence of *H. nana* in human tissues. Most infections by the dwarf tapeworm are asymptomatic. Autoinfection or infection with a heavy worm load is associated with abdominal pain, headache, diarrhea and anorexia.

### 3. Laboratory Diagnosis

Diagnosis rests on the demonstration of the typical *H. nana* eggs with their six-hooked embryos and polar filaments.

### 4. Treatment and Prevention

Praziquantel or niclosamide are effective against *H. nana*. Prevention requires proper treatment and disposal of fecal material accompanied by good personal hygiene.

## VIII. PLATYHELMINTHES (FLATWORMS)— TREMATODES

### A. *Trematodes: Schistosoma mansoni, S. japonicum, S. haematobium*

#### 1. Transmission and Life Cycle

Trematodes or flukes have one deep sucker around the oral cavity and another one the ventral side of the fluke, and they serve as organs of host cell attachment and movement. They have a primitive digestive system, a nervous and excretory system and, with the exception of schistosomes, are leaf-like and hermaphroditic. Schistosomes differ in that they possess genital organs of both sexes and their bodies are closely similar to those of roundworms. Also, the ova produced by the fertilized female schistosomes are non-operculated (see Fig. 6-10). The ova of *S. mansoni* have a distinct lateral spine, *S. japonicum* eggs have a rudimentary lateral spine and the ova of *S. haematobium* possess a prominent terminal spine. In the life cycle of schistosomes, the eggs are passed in the human stools, and

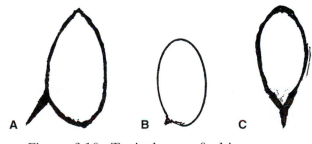

Figure 6-10. Typical eggs of schistosomes:
(**A**) *S. mansoni;* (**B**) *S. japonicum;*
(**C**) *S. haematobium.*

when they reach water either hatch immediately or mature before they release swimming miracidium. This is ingested by a snail that serves as intermediate host for schistosomes. The miracidia undergo asexual multiplication within snails, and cercariae are produced. Cercariae seek a second intermediate host, such as freshwater fish, crab, crayfish or a plant, and transform to metacercariae. Humans acquire schistosomiasis when free-swimming cercariae or metacercariae penetrate the human skin, migrate to their destination and become adult flukes.

## 2. Pathogenesis and Clinical Manifestations

Ova of *S. mansoni* and *S. japonicum* damage the walls of inferior and superior mesenteric venules of the small and large intestines. Eggs of *S. haematobium* produce fibrosis and granulomas in the wall of the bladder, which may lead to carcinoma of the bladder. The tissue damage is due to production of oval proteolytic enzymes and to the host inflammatory responses. Schistosomes evade host immune responses by coating their surface with host antigens to which the immune system does not normally respond. Most initial infections are asymptomatic. However, chronic infections may be associated with dermatitis, eosinophilia, elevated IgE serum levels, sensitization to oval antigens, fever, lymphadenopathy, hepatitis, diarrhea, dysentery, incontinence, bladder or lung hemorrhage, fibrosis of damaged tissue, granuloma and pseudotubercle formation.

## 3. Laboratory Diagnosis

Diagnosis of schistosomiasis requires the demonstration of typical ova of schistosomes in the stools or urine of patients.

## 4. Treatment and Prevention

Praziquantel is the drug of choice for the treatment of schistosomiasis. Prevention can only be partially successful and involves such measures as proper disposal of fecal material and urine, use of molluscicides and mass chemotherapy of populations.

## B. *Paragonimus westermani* (Lung Fluke)

### 1. Transmission and Life Cycle

*P. westermani* is a reddish brown, short, plump (10 by 5 mm), hermaphroditic fluke found encapsulated in the lung parenchyma. The lung trematode produces golden-brown, operculated ova with a distinct peri-opercular shoulder which are passed in the stools. Paragonomiasis is acquired by the ingestion of metacercariae in crayfish or freshwater crabs that serve as the second intermediate hosts. The life cycle of *P. westermani* is similar to schistosomes except that this trematode is found encapsulated in the lung parenchyma.

### 2. Pathogenesis and Clinical Manifestations

The pathogenesis and symptomatology of paragonomiasis resemble that of schistosomiasis. The key clinical feature of paragonomiasis is chronic cough with bloody sputum. Thus, infection with *P. westermani* has to be differentiated from tuberculosis.

### 3. Laboratory Diagnosis

Diagnosis of paragonomiasis requires the demonstration of the typical ova of *P. westermani* in the stool or sputum of patients.

### 4. Treatment and Prevention

Praziquantel or bithionol is effective against the lung fluke.
Prevention requires thorough cooking of shellfish before ingestion.

## C. *Clonorchis sinensis* (Chinese Liver Fluke)

### 1. Transmission and Life Cycle

*C. sinensis* is a flat, leaf-like, grayish fluke that tapers anteriorly and is rounded posteriorly. It has oral and ventral suckers, and its ova are light yellowish-brown with a convex operculum at the smaller end. The Chinese liver fluke is hermaphroditic. Clonorchiasis is acquired by the ingestion of metacercariae in raw, poorly cooked, smoked or pickled fish. The life cycle of *C. sinensis* is similar to schistosomes except that the immature liver flukes mature in the biliary ducts.

### 2. Pathogenesis and Clinical Manifestations

The mechanism of pathogenicity and symptomatology of clonorchiasis resemble that of schistosomiasis.

### 3. Laboratory Diagnosis

Clonorchiasis can be diagnosed by the demonstration of small, yellowish-brown eggs of *C. sinensis* in the stool or in duodenal aspirates from patients.

### 4. Treatment and Prevention

Praziquantel is used for the treatment of clonorchiasis.
Prevention demands thorough cooking or sanitary preparation of smoked or pickled freshwater fish and proper disposal of human feces.

## D. *Fasciola hepatica* (Liver Fluke)

### 1. Transmission and Life Cycle

*F. hepatica* is a large (30 by 13 mm), broad, flat, leaf-like trematode with a prominent anterior cone and a branching of the intestinal ceca that is used to differentiate it from *Fasciolopsis buski*. The adult liver flukes live in the biliary tract, are hermaphroditic and produce very large (130–150 µm), symmetrical, operculated ova. Humans are infected with *F. hepatica* by eating watercress and other vegetables contaminated with encysted metacercariae. In other respects, the life cycle of *F. hepatica* is similar to that of schistosomes.

### 2. Pathogenesis and Clinical Manifestations

The pathogenesis and symptomatology of *F. hepatica* are very similar to that of schistosomiasis. In variance with other liver flukes, this trematode does not tend to induce cholangiocarcinoma.

### 3. Laboratory Diagnosis

Definitive diagnosis is based on the detection of typical ova of *F. hepatica* in the feces of patients and by serological tests.

### 4. Treatment and Prevention

Bithionol is the drug of choice. Abendazole or triclabendazole may be used as alternative drugs. Surgical intervention is used to remove adult worms from the larynx and pharynx. Prevention of infection by *F. hepatica* is difficult but may be minimized by not eating salads containing watercress or other freshwater vegetables.

## E. *Fasciolopsis buski* (Intestinal Fluke)

*F. buski* is similar to *F. hepatica* except that the adult worms live in the intestine and not in the biliary tract.

# Bibliography

Braunwald E, Fauci AS, Kasper DL, et al. *Harrison's Principles of Internal Medicine,* 15th ed. New York: McGraw-Hill; 2001.

Levinson WE, Jawetz E. *Medical Microbiology and Immunology,* 7th ed. New York: McGraw-Hill; 2002.

Murray PR, Rosenthal KS, Kobayashi GS, Pfaller MA. *Medical Microbiology,* 4th ed. St. Louis, MO: Mosby; 2002.

Roitt IM, Delves PJ. *Roitt's Essentials of Immunology,* 10th ed. London, UK: Blackwell Science Ltd; 2001.

Yotis WW, Friedman H. *Appleton & Lange's Review of Microbiology & Immunology,* 4th ed. New York: McGraw-Hill; 2001.

# Index

*Note:* Page numbers followed by *f* or *t* indicate figures and tables, respectively.